Awesome Foods for Active Kids

ORDERING

Trade bookstores in the U.S. and Canada please contact:

Publishers Group West
1700 Fourth Street, Berkeley CA 94710
Phone: (800) 788-3123   Fax: (510) 528-3444

Hunter House books are available at bulk discounts for textbook course
adoptions; to qualifying community, health-care, and government organizations;
and for special promotions and fund-raising. For details please contact:

Special Sales Department
Hunter House Inc., PO Box 2914, Alameda CA 94501-0914
Phone: (510) 865-5282   Fax: (510) 865-4295
E-mail: ordering@hunterhouse.com

Individuals can order our books from most bookstores, by calling (800) 266-5592,
or from our website at **www.hunterhouse.com**

PROJECT CREDITS
Cover Design: Peri Poloni
Recipe Editor: Sue Spitler
Nutritional Consultant: Linda Yoakam, M.S., R.D., L.D.
Copy Editor: Kelley Blewster
Indexers: Robert and Cynthia Swanson
Acquisitions Editor: Jeanne Brondino
Editor: Alexandra Mummery
Publishing Assistant: Herman Leung
Office Assistant: Joe Winebarger
Publicist: Jillian Steinberger
Publishing Intern: Shelley McGuire
Customer Service Manager: Christina Sverdrup
Order Fulfillment: Washul Lakdhon
Administrator: Theresa Nelson
Computer Support: Peter Eichelberger
Publisher: Kiran S. Rana

Manufactured in Canada by Transcontinental Printing

9 8 7 6 5 4 3 2 1   First Edition   06 07 08 09 10

Awesome Foods for Active Kids

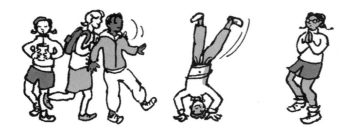

THE ABCS OF EATING FOR ENERGY AND HEALTH

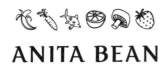

ANITA BEAN

Hunter House
PUBLISHERS

LIBRARY OF CONGRESS CATALOGING-IN-PUBLICATION DATA
Bean, Anita.
    Awesome foods for active kids : the ABCs of eating for energy and health / Anita Bean.
        p. cm.
    "First published 2002 by A & C Black Publishers Ltd, London."
    Summary: "Information and suggestions for parents who want to ensure their active children
(ages 5 to 16) are getting a healthy diet, including over 80 vegetarian and non-vegetarian recipes with
nutrition analysis"—Provided by publisher.
    Includes bibliographical references and index.
    ISBN-13: 978-0-89793-475-6 (pbk.)
    ISBN-10: 0-89793-475-X (pbk.)
    1. Children—Nutrition. 2. Children—Health and hygiene. I. Title.
RJ206.B43 2005
618.92'39—dc22   2005013625

Contents

Acknowledgments   ix

Introduction   1

CHAPTER 1: *Kids' Food and Health*   5
   Does It Matter What Children Eat?
   How Do Kids' Diets Measure Up?
   Why Should You Change What Children Eat?
   So How Can I Influence Children's Eating Habits?
   Television and Advertising
   How Can You Combat Advertising Pressure?
   Looking at the Labels
   What to Avoid

CHAPTER 2: *What Should Active Children Eat?*   14
   How Does the Food Pyramid Work?
   How Many Servings?
   How Big Is a Portion?
   Building the Pyramid
   Looking after Children's Teeth

CHAPTER 3: *Protein Power*   25
   What Happens to Protein in the Body?
   Will Extra Protein Make Stronger Muscles?
   How Much Protein?
   How to Get Enough Protein
   What about Vegetarian Diets?
   What about Protein Supplements?

CHAPTER 4: *Carb-Charging*   30
Why Do Kids Need Carbs?
How Much Carbohydrate?
Which Types of Carbohydrate Are Best?
Carbohydrates and the Glycemic Index

CHAPTER 5: *Fat Matters*   37
Why Is Fat Needed?
What's the Difference Between Saturated and Unsaturated Fats?
What Are the Essential Fats?
What Is Hydrogenated Fat?
How Much Fat Should Children Eat?

CHAPTER 6: *Vitamins and Minerals*   43
What Do Vitamins and Minerals Do?
How to Get Enough Vitamins and Minerals
How Can You Get Children to Eat More Fruits and Vegetables?
Guide to Vitamins and Minerals
Do Active Children Need More Vitamins and Minerals?
Should Children Take Vitamin Supplements?
Phytochemicals
Antioxidants

CHAPTER 7: *Eating for Action*   59
How Much Food Should My Child Eat?
What Should Children Eat Before Training or Competition?
Timing the Pre-Exercise Meal
Eating Before an Event
What Should Children Eat During Exercise?
What Should Children Eat after Exercise?
Traveling and Competing Away from Home

CHAPTER 8: *Drinking for Action*   70
Why Is Drinking Important for My Child?
Dehydration Check-Up
How Much Should Children Drink?
How to Fit It All In
How to Make Children Drink while Exercising
What Should Children Drink?

CHAPTER 9: *Overweight Kids* 78

What Are the Dangers for Children of Being Overweight?

Heart Symptoms in Obese Children

How Can I Tell If a Child Is Overweight?

Why Do Children Become Overweight?

How Should I Deal with Children's Weight Problems?

What Practical Help Can I Give?

How Can Children Be Encouraged to Be More Active?

How Much Exercise Should Children Get?

How Much Exercise Do Children Really Get?

How Can Children Adopt Healthier Eating Habits?

How Can I Avoid Mealtimes Becoming a Battleground?

Should Children Lose Weight for Sports?

How Can I Discourage Television Viewing?

CHAPTER 10: *Underweight Kids and Fussy Eaters* 93

Thin or Underweight?

Why Are Some Children Thin?

Feeding Children with Small Appetites

Feeding Fussy Eaters

Feeding Very Active Children

Strength Training for Children

CHAPTER 11: *Eating at School* 102

Packing a Healthy Lunch

What's in School Meals?

What Should I Encourage Children to Eat for School Lunch?

What Can I Give Children after School?

CHAPTER 12: *Eating Disorders* 113

What Are Eating Disorders?

What Are the Causes of Eating Disorders?

Why Are Eating Disorders Common among Young Athletes?

How Do I Know If a Child Has an Eating Disorder?

How Will an Eating Disorder Affect a Child's Health
    and Performance?

What Can I Do If I Think a Child Has an Eating Disorder?

Preventing Eating Disorders

CHAPTER 13: *Kids' Menu Plans*   120

CHAPTER 14: *Main Meals*   131

CHAPTER 15: *Meatless Main Meals*   145

CHAPTER 16: *Salads*   159
  Salad Dressings

CHAPTER 17: *Super Soups*   164

CHAPTER 18: *Fast Food*   170

CHAPTER 19: *And to Finish*   184

CHAPTER 20: *Kids' Snacks*   193

CHAPTER 21: *Delicious Drinks*   202

Notes   207

Resources   209
  Online Resources
  Useful Addresses
  Recommended Reading

Index   211

Acknowledgments

The author, Anita Bean, her husband, Simon, and their daughters, Lucy, 4, and Chloe, 6.

I would like to thank my husband, Simon, for all his support during the writing of this book, and my two wonderful daughters, Chloe and Lucy, for giving me the inspiration to put pen to paper, and also for eating (or at least trying) the recipes in this book.

IMPORTANT NOTE

The material in this book is intended to provide a review of information regarding nutrition for children. Every effort has been made to provide accurate and dependable information. The contents of this book have been compiled through professional research and in consultation with medical professionals. However, professionals in the field may have differing opinions, and change is always taking place.

Therefore, the publisher, author, and editors, as well as the professionals quoted in the book cannot be held responsible for any error, omission, or dated material. The author and publisher assume no responsibility for any outcome of applying the information in this book in a program of self-care or under the care of a licensed practitioner. If you have questions concerning your or your child's nutrition or diet, or about the application of the information described in this book, consult a qualified health-care professional.

Introduction

This book is for everyone who cares about what children eat. Whether you have children of your own, teach them, or look after them, you need to know what they should be eating so they will achieve great health and peak performance.

How can you get children to eat food that tastes good, does them good, and helps them perform better? Children only eat food they like. If they don't like the taste of it, they won't eat it, no matter how nutritious it may be. But that doesn't mean succumbing to a diet of artificially flavored, highly sweetened, fat-laden processed food, or existing on fast food and "kid's meals." Children are perfectly capable of appreciating the taste of healthy foods if you know how to present them—and if you keep on presenting them! You also need to set a good example yourself. Children are more likely to do what you do, not what you merely say. So, if they see you enjoying healthy meals and taking part in regular physical activity, they are more likely to do the same. You can't expect them to eat healthily or to get regular exercise if they see you eating candy and cookies, watching TV all the time, and taking the car everywhere!

Clearly, the earlier you can help kids establish good eating and exercise habits, the more likely they will enjoy a lifetime of good health. My two children don't think twice about walking to school every day, cycling to their after-school activities instead of being driven, and snacking on fruit instead of sweets. They have never known anything different, and they have seen both of their parents doing the same.

Awesome Foods for Active Kids: The ABCs of Eating for Energy and Health explains what active children should be eating and offers practical suggestions for healthy meals, snacks, and drinks. Unlike other books on kids' nutrition, it emphasizes the importance of activity and sports. Whether they're playing in the park, learning to swim, or taking part in organized athletics, children will perform better by eating and drinking the right foods. I have witnessed the transformation in children's energy levels and physical performance when they kick unhealthy eating habits and start to eat balanced meals. They have more energy, they suffer fewer colds and minor infections, they have clearer skin and brighter eyes, and their powers of concentration at school dramatically increase.

Of course, it's not always easy to persuade children to eat healthily. It's difficult to combat the pressures of advertising by manufacturers trying to sell you fatty, sugary foods disguised as children's food. Then there's pester power from your kids to buy foods sporting their favorite cartoon characters and foods their friends eat. Believe me, I've heard it all from my own children!

Everyone hates the thought of wasting food, so it's easy to get into the routine of giving children only those foods you know they will eat. Time pressures also mean that it's easier to reach for packages and jars than to make meals from scratch. The trouble with falling into this pattern is that children end up eating only a small range of foods and may miss out on important nutrients and exciting flavors. Many of my friends complain that they often get stuck for inspiration and are in desperate need of fresh mealtime ideas. Message received! Chapters 13 through 21 of this book contain four weekly menu plans plus lots of healthy recipes that are easy to prepare. They have all been tested by willing—and hungry—volunteers. Only those that passed the child-approval test were included.

Results from the 1999–2000 National Health and Nutrition Examination Survey (NHANES) indicate that an estimated 15 percent of U.S. children and adolescents ages six to nineteen are overweight.[1] Compare this to the same statistics from the early 1970s, when only 4 percent of kids and 6 percent of adolescents in the U.S. were overweight. These statistics reinforce the fact that children need to be encouraged to become more active, spend less time doing sedentary activities, and eat more healthily. At the other end of the scale, some children eat very little and cause a lot of concern to their parents. In this book I give suggestions for dealing with overweight kids, picky eaters, and underweight kids. I also present information about eating disorders and about what you can do to help someone suspected of having anorexia or bulimia. Prevention of the poor self-image that plays a key role in eating disorders is always the ideal, so I have drawn up a checklist of points for fostering a positive body image in children.

As you will see, *Awesome Foods for Active Kids* covers a vast range of nutrition and fitness issues relevant to children. I have combined scientific evidence, recommendations from authoritative experts, and information from surveys with practical sense and my own experience as a sports nutritionist and mother. I hope you will find the book useful and inspirational, and that you and your children will enjoy fabulous food and great health!

– Anita

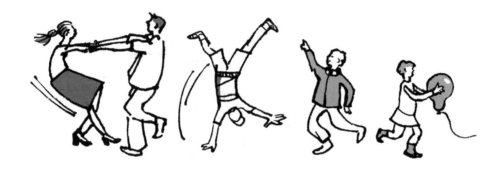

CHAPTER 1

Kids' Food and Health

The food you feed your children will affect their health now and in the future. It also determines their energy levels, their physical performance, and their success in sports and recreational activities. Their brains, too, are hungry for energy and nutrients, so a healthy diet is vital for optimizing their mental performance. Teaching children to enjoy a nutritious, varied diet will help them to grow up healthy, fit, and full of energy.

Here are just a few of the benefits your children will get from improving their diet. They will

- have more energy and zest
- do better in sports and games
- feel brighter and more alert
- concentrate more easily on schoolwork
- sleep well and wake up feeling refreshed
- have fewer illnesses
- have clearer skin, brighter eyes, and shiny hair

Does It Matter What Children Eat?

Many parents think it doesn't matter too much what their kids eat, in the belief that their children will soon grow out of unhealthy eating habits. I've seen moms give in to demands for less nutritious food such as sweets and chips because "they're skinny so it doesn't matter what they eat," or because "eating something is better than eating nothing.' " Parents have frequently said to me, "My kids are growing okay and still running around, so their diet can't be too bad." Wrong on all counts!

The truth is that children's eating habits do not automatically improve as they get older; they nearly always get worse. Children continue eating only what they are accustomed to. A bad diet now means a bad diet in five or ten years. The sooner you start to teach children how to eat healthily, the better. By changing their diet now and helping them to become more active you will increase their chances of enjoying better health now and in the future.

Children need lots of nutrients to make sure they grow and develop properly. The biggest problem with "junk" food is that it displaces foods that provide important vitamins and minerals. A child who fills up on a chocolate bar has missed out on eating a piece of fresh fruit or yogurt or a sandwich–foods that supply a lot more nutrients than sweets do.

So what about their growth? Even if children appear to be growing normally in height, that does not mean they are as healthy and fit as they could be. In fact, a child would have to be severely malnourished for his or her growth to suffer, so don't judge children's diets according to whether they are growing. There are many other indicators of poor eating habits. Take the quiz below to find out whether you should change your child's eating habits:

QUESTIONNAIRE
Do You Need to Change Your Children's Eating Habits?

1. Is your child frequently tired and lethargic? ☐

2. Does your child tire easily during physical play or sports? ☐

3. Is your child often pale? ☐

4. Do your child's eyes look dull? ☐

5. Is your child's hair very fine, dry, or brittle? ☐

6. Does your child often have difficulty getting out of bed in the morning? ☐

7. Does your child suffer frequent colds, coughs, and infections? ☐

8. Is your child noticeably fatter than other children of the same age? ☐

9. Is your child constipated? ☐

10. Is your child noticeably thinner or smaller than other children of the same age? ☐

11. Does your child suffer frequent loose bowel movements? ☐

12. Is your child prone to stomachaches, nausea, or sickness? ☐

13. Does your child often have difficulty concentrating? ☐

14. Does your child have mood swings? ☐

15. Is your child often irritable or restless? ☐

If you checked eight or more boxes you definitely need to help your child adopt healthier eating habits.

If you checked between four and eight boxes your child would probably benefit from a healthier diet.

If you checked fewer than four boxes your child's diet may be adequate; but is there room for improvement?

IMPORTANT NOTE: This questionnaire is not intended to diagnose or treat any illness or underlying medical condition. You should always check with your doctor if you suspect your child may have an allergy, infection, or medical condition.

How Do Kids' Diets Measure Up?

Snacking, grazing, and eating on the run are the norm for many children as our culture moves away from regular mealtimes. According to a U.S.-government study of about five thousand children ages two to eighteen, the vast majority of American children eat a diet that is poor and needs improvement. As kids get older, their diets worsen; whereas 35 percent of children ages two and three have a "good" overall diet, only about 5 percent of teenagers do. (The study assessed how diets stacked up against ten components, cumulatively labeled the Healthy Eating Index.) Specifically:

- Of kids age four and older, fewer than 30 percent ate the recommended number of servings of fruits per day, and fewer than 40 percent ate the recommended number of servings of vegetables per day (the number of recommended servings is a minimum of two fruits and three vegetables).

- Sixty percent or more of children ages two to eighteen consumed more fat than is recommended (the amount recommended is no more than 30 percent of total calories).

- Over 60 percent of children age seven and over consumed more sodium than the recommended 2,400 milligrams (mg) or less per day.

- More than half of all children over age three failed to eat the recommended number of servings of *any* of the five major food groups (grains, dairy, meat, veggies, and fruit).[2]

Although the Healthy Eating Index didn't measure sugar consumption, it's very likely that in place of all the healthy foods kids are *not* eating, they're consuming excessive amounts of candy, cookies, cakes, pastries, soda pop, and other sugary snacks. It's when these poor eating habits are coupled with inactivity–watching television, playing computer games, and getting around by car all the time–that the trouble really begins. Too many calories and too little exercise will cause an unhealthy increase in their body fat.

Why Should You Change What Children Eat?

What children eat now influences their future eating habits. If they eat a healthy diet now, and participate in physical activity from an early age, they are more likely to remain healthy and active during adulthood. Children who are used to eating vegetables or walking to school every day (even when it rains) will continue to eat healthy food and to regard physical activity as an integral part of their life. Equally, those who graze on a diet of fast foods and salty snacks and spend hours glued to the television are setting themselves up for a lifetime of poor eating habits and inactivity. What's certain is that unhealthy eating and activity habits are harder to undo in later life.

It's also important to realize that the seeds of certain illnesses such as

coronary heart disease and diabetes are sown during childhood. Some overweight children as young as ten years old show signs of artery damage and
suffer from high blood pressure.[3] The good news is that changing children's
diets and encouraging them to be more active can prevent health problems
in the future. Now is the time to teach children healthy eating and exercise
habits.

So How Can I Influence Children's Eating Habits?

Children are more likely to do as you do. Being a good role model will encourage good habits in the kids who spend time with you. If children see
you enjoying eating healthy foods and getting regular exercise, they are likely
to do the same. It's important to realize that attitudes toward food, weight,
and exercise are established early on. Most eating behavior is learned.

What children see and eat at home makes a big impact on their lifelong
dietary and exercise habits. Eating a lot of high-fat, salty, or sugary foods
conditions a child's tastes to those types of foods. Unless you make an effort
to introduce fresh, whole foods into their diets, children will continue to
choose bland, processed foods and to reject fresh foods such as fruit or vegetables, even though fresh food has stronger flavors. You can't blame them for
choosing and eating what they are accustomed to.

Television and Advertising

Children are encouraged to eat a poor diet by television advertising. Surveys
have found that 95 percent of the food advertisements broadcast during children's prime-time television is for foods with high levels of fat, sugar, and/or
salt (e.g., chocolate, chips, sweetened breakfast cereals, fast-food restaurants).[4] This creates a conflict between the types of foods promoted by ad-
vertisers and those recommended by the government. Moreover, it increases
children's "pester power" as children nag their parents to buy particular
products. Since no controls exist over the types of foods and drinks featured
on children's TV, the best action you can take is to set sensible limits on how
much TV your children can watch (see the section in Chapter 9 titled "How
Can I Discourage Television Viewing?")

How Can You Combat Advertising Pressure?

Manufacturers use lots of tricks to persuade you to buy foods and drinks that are unhealthy for children. Here are the major sneaky promotions used and some suggestions about what you can do to combat them.

CARTOON CHARACTERS ON FOOD PACKAGES

These are designed to grab children's attention. Many of these types of products are unhealthy and consist of low-quality ingredients.

What you can do: Don't encourage your children to choose which product they want. Learn how to read the label (see page 000). Explain that the food inside is very sugary/fatty/salty.

PROMOTIONS ON THE PACKAGING

Products that contain collectable free gifts or cheap offers for toys and gadgets will appeal to children.

What you can do: Look carefully at what's in the product before you agree to buy it. If it's a product that you would rather not buy, stand firm and steer your children towards healthier choices.

INTRODUCING LOYALTY

By encouraging the collection of product labels or box tops for schoolbooks, computer equipment, and membership to clubs, or by providing interactive websites, food manufacturers encourage brand loyalty. This is fine if it's a healthy product; otherwise the ploy pressures parents to buy products they wouldn't otherwise want for their children.

What you can do: Point out to your child that saving labels is usually tiresome and time-consuming and offers poor value for the money spent.

NOVELTY VALUE

Children love novelty shapes and colors, "mini" food sizes, new textures, and anything that makes a product easy and fun to eat. That's great if it's a healthy product–such as fun-sized cheese portions–but many novelty products are high in sugar, fat, or salt (as well as being expensive).

What you can do: Make your own healthy novelty foods. Chop vegetables or fruit into fun shapes, serve food in fun dishes, and place healthy snacks like nuts in tiny pots.

ADDED VITAMINS

By adding extra vitamins to a basically unhealthy product, such as a sugary drink, a sugary processed cereal, or a packet of sweets, manufacturers know that parents are more likely to buy it. But this doesn't turn an inherently unhealthy product into a good one. Vitamin-enriched sweets or cookies are still high in sugar and bad for children's teeth.

What you can do: If you wouldn't buy the product without the added vitamins, don't buy it with them.

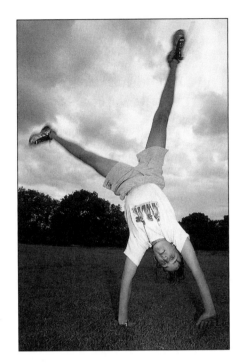

Looking at the Labels

To judge the quality of the food you buy for your children, look at the Nutrition Facts panel on food packages. Use the table below to help you determine if the food contains unhealthy amounts of fat, sugar, or salt (sodium).

Amount per 100 grams (or per serving if larger than 100 grams)		
	THIS IS A LOT	**THIS IS A LITTLE**
Total fat	20 g	3 g
Saturated fat	5 g	1 g
Sugar	10 g	3 g
Sodium	500 mg	100 mg

What to Avoid[5]

If you know what to look for, studying the labels can also help you determine whether the food you're considering contains any of the following substances, which are to be avoided.

ARTIFICIAL ADDITIVES

Additives are supposed to be safe in theory. But they may provoke an allergic reaction or a similar adverse reaction in some children. Because artificial additives are found in so many children's foods (up to three-quarters of children's foods contains additives, according to one survey by the natural-foods company Organix), children could consume huge amounts of additives by the time they reach their teens.[6] Sweets, savory snacks, desserts, and snack bars are the worst offenders, so make sure that the only additives in the products you buy are natural ones, such as vanilla extract.

HIDDEN SUGAR

Look out for sucrose, glucose syrup, dextrose, fruit syrup, glucose—they all mean sugar. The two main problems with sugar are that it damages children's teeth and increases their risk for diabetes. (In the United States, type-II diabetes, traditionally known as "adult-onset diabetes," is now being diagnosed in record numbers among children and adolescents, a fact directly attributable to lifestyle factors such as increased rates of obesity and physical inactivity.)[7]

ARTIFICIAL SWEETENERS

Aspartame, acesulfame K, and saccharin are common in both "sugar-free"

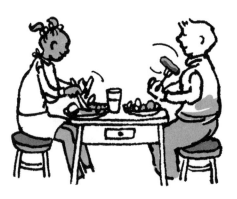

and ordinary versions of foods and drinks. They may not rot children's teeth, but they perpetuate a liking for intense sweetness. Whether they are really safe for children is still a controversial issue.

HYDROGENATED FAT

Check labels for both hydrogenated and partially hydrogenated fats in margarines, pastries, pies, cakes, ice cream, desserts, cookies, chocolate-coated bars, cereal bars, crackers, and chips. Solidifying cheap liquid oils produces this type of manmade fat. The problem is that the process also creates trans fats (see page 40), which are even more harmful to health than saturated fats. They increase the levels of "bad" fats in the blood and reduce the levels of "good" fats.

Tips for Changing Your Family's Eating Behavior

- Explain the benefits of eating more healthily (see above). Present them in terms your children can understand and directly relate to, e.g., having more energy to play soccer; feeling more refreshed in the morning.

- Put children in control of some of their food choices, e.g., allow them to choose which vegetables to eat; let them suggest a new meal.

- Set some realistic goals, e.g., to eat two pieces of fruit a day; to try a new vegetable; to replace chips with an apple or a handful of nuts.

- Set up a reward system, e.g., award a star or sticker for each healthy eating behavior. When, say, ten stars have been earned, choose a reward (preferably nonfood, such as a new toy or a special trip) that has been agreed upon in advance.

- Increase the range of foods in your family's repertoire; try new recipes and offer new snacks (see recipes on pages 131–206).

- Set a good example yourself; don't show reservation in trying new foods.

- Praise children for trying a new food. Even if they don't like it, encourage them to explain why. Use the motto "Taste before you judge"—it always works with my children, who end up eating all of it!

- If a new food or dish is rejected initially, leave it out for a while, then reintroduce it a week or so later. Children will eventually like healthy foods if they are continually exposed to them.

CHAPTER 2

What Should Active Children Eat?

All children need to eat a balanced diet to ensure proper growth, good health, and physical activity. For active children, eating the right foods is especially important for their performance and recovery during and after sports. So, how do you set about planning healthy meals for children? This chapter provides a practical guide to meal planning based on the Food Pyramid.

How Does the Food Pyramid Work?

The Food Pyramid, shown on page ooo, is designed to meet the nutritional needs of active children, and makes planning a balanced diet for children easier. It is adapted from the U.S. Department of Agriculture's Food Guide Pyramid and the British Health Department Agency's National Food Guide. The British guide includes only five food groups. This Food Pyramid bumps that number up to the following seven, more finely tuned to the needs of active children: grains, vegetables, fruit, dairy, protein-rich foods, essential fats, and sugary and fatty foods. Each group provides some, but not all, of the nutrients and energy children need. The pyramid gives you a visual guide to the proportion of different foods that make up a balanced diet. The lower the layer, the more foods children need from that group for a healthy diet. Thus, the foods in the bottom layer—grains—should form the bulk of children's diet. The next layer—fruit and vegetables—should be the next most prominent in a child's diet, followed by protein-rich foods and dairy foods. Finally, the foods at the very top of the pyramid—fatty and sugary foods—have a lot of calories from fat and sugars and should be eaten only in small amounts. There are no forbidden foods in the pyramid. Variety and moderation are the most important principles when it comes to putting together a healthy eating plan. Here's how to use the pyramid:

- Include foods from each group in the pyramid each day
- Make sure you include a variety of foods within each group
- Aim to have the recommended number of servings each day
- Check the serving sizes given below

How Many Servings?

Aim to include the suggested number of servings of each food group daily (see table below). Remember, these are guidelines, and on some days children may need more or less of a certain food group.

Recommended Servings for Each Food Group	
FOOD GROUP	**NUMBER OF SERVINGS**
Grains	6–8
Vegetables	3
Fruit	2
Dairy	2–3
Protein-rich foods	2–3
Essential fats and oils	1
Sugary and fatty foods	1 or less

How Big Is a Portion?

Of course, the exact amount of each food a child needs varies, depending on his or her age, size, and activity level. In general, younger children need fewer calories than older children, so offer them smaller amounts. Their appetites also vary from one day to the next, and you'll find that on some days

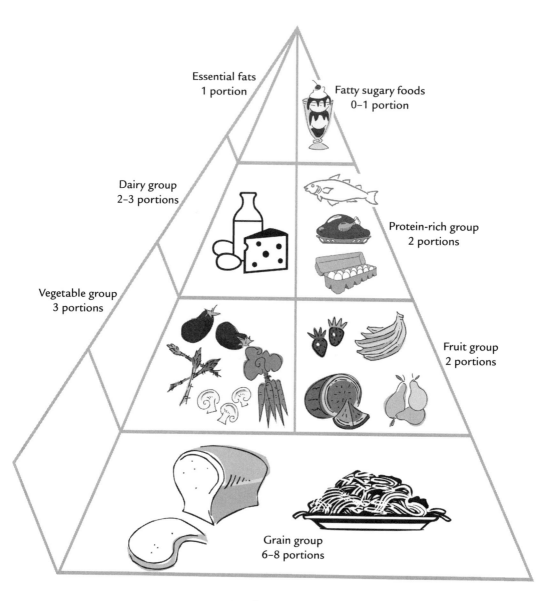

Food Pyramid

they eat much bigger portions than on others. That's fine; for the most part you should be guided by your children's appetites. Remember, it is the overall balance of foods that is most important. The following section gives a guide to suitable portion sizes.

Building the Pyramid

GRAINS AND POTATOES

This group includes bread, pasta, rice, noodles, breakfast cereals, oatmeal, and crackers, as well as starchy vegetables such as potatoes, sweet potatoes, parsnips, and yams. These foods provide complex carbohydrates (starch and fiber) for energy, B vitamins, and various minerals including iron. A typical child serving size is:

	5–10 YEARS	11–15 YEARS
Bread	1 small slice	1 large slice
Rolls, muffins, bagels	½ large roll	1 large roll
Pasta or rice	3 tablespoons	4 tablespoons
Oatmeal, hot cereal	3 tablespoons	4 tablespoons
Breakfast cereal	3 tablespoons	4 tablespoons
Potatoes, sweet potatoes, yams	1 small (about the size of an egg)	1 medium (about the size of the child's fist)
Crackers	2	3

Six servings in a day can be achieved by eating

- a bowl of breakfast cereal (2 servings, if child eats ½ cup of cereal)
- a slice of toast as a snack
- a baked potato for lunch
- two crackers as a snack
- a pasta or rice dish for supper

FRUITS AND VEGETABLES

Fruits and vegetables are rich in vitamins and minerals, and are also great sources of fiber and phytochemicals, which help protect the body from disease and boost immunity. Offer as many different types of fruit and vegetables in your children's diet as possible. Mix colors—yellow, orange, red, green—so they will get a good balance of vitamins and phytochemicals. Each day, try to include at least one green leafy vegetable such as broccoli or cabbage, and one yellow-orange vegetable such as carrots. Offer a variety of fruit, too, including yellow-orange fruit such as peaches or satsuma mandarins, berries such as strawberries or blackberries, and tree fruit such as apples or pears. A typical child portion is:

	5–10 YEARS	11–15 YEARS
Cooked vegetables	2 tablespoons	3 tablespoons
Raw vegetables, e.g., carrots, pepper, cucumber sticks	2 tablespoons	3 tablespoons
Tomatoes	1 medium or 3 cherry tomatoes	2 medium or 6 cherry tomatoes
Apples, pears, oranges, peaches, bananas	1 small piece of fruit	1 medium piece of fruit
Berries, e.g., strawberries, blackberries, raspberries	2 tablespoons	3 tablespoons
Small fruit, e.g., kiwi fruit, satsumas, plums, apricots	1 piece of fruit	2 pieces of fruit

Five portions a day can be achieved by eating

- an apple or kiwi fruit as a snack
- crudités or vegetable soup for lunch
- cauliflower with cheese sauce and carrots for supper
- fruit crumble or fruit salad for dessert

DAIRY FOODS

The foods in this group—milk, cheese, yogurt, and cottage cheese—are rich in calcium, which is important for children's growing bones. They also provide protein and several of the B vitamins. Full-fat products also contribute fat (mainly saturated) and the fat-soluble vitamins A and D. You can reduce fat easily by switching to reduced-fat products, such as low-fat milk or yogurt. Low-fat products are suitable for children over five years old. A typical child portion is:

	5–10 YEARS	11–15 YEARS
Milk	1 small cup or glass	1 medium cup or glass
Yogurt or cottage cheese	1 carton (8 oz.)	1 carton (8 oz.)
Hard cheese	2 slices (1½ oz.)	2 slices (1½ oz.)

Two servings a day can be achieved by eating

- breakfast cereal with milk (½ serving)
- baked potato with a slice of cheese (½ serving)
- 1 carton of yogurt (1 serving)

PROTEIN-RICH FOODS

The foods in this group include lean meat, such as beef and lamb (trimmed of fat), chicken, turkey, fish, eggs, beans, lentils, nuts, soy, and meat substitutes, such as Quorn (a product recently introduced in the United states that is made from mycoprotein, the same protein contained in mushrooms). They supply protein as well as several vitamins and minerals. Limit high-fat meats, sausages, burgers, and "nuggets" to no more than three portions a week because they contain a lot of saturated fat and harmful trans fats (see page 39), not to mention various artificial additives. These fast "kiddie" foods may appear to be a good solution to mealtime dilemmas when you are rushed, but

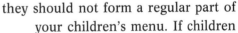

they should not form a regular part of your children's menu. If children only eat burgers, nuggets, and fish sticks, when are they going to learn how to appreciate proper food? The less you rely on these ready-made fat-laden foods, the better it will be for your children's palates and health.

WHAT ABOUT VEGETARIANS?

Vegetarians get plenty of protein from plant sources, such as beans, lentils, and soy products (see page 27). In addition, you may substitute extra dairy foods for one of the portions in this group, as dairy foods are also rich in protein. For example, children may have three portions of dairy foods and one portion of protein-rich foods. However, do not eliminate the protein group entirely, as these foods supply valuable vitamins and minerals lacking in dairy foods.

Even if your family is not vegetarian, try to introduce some vegetable-protein foods such as beans, lentils, and soy products into your children's diet. These foods provide a unique type of fiber that's particularly beneficial for the digestive system, as well as lots of important minerals and phytochemicals absent from animal proteins.

All children should aim to have about half of their servings of this group from nonmeat sources.

A typical child portion is:

	5–10 YEARS	11–15 YEARS
Lean meat	1 slice	1–2 slices
Chicken or turkey	2 thin slices	2 medium slices
Fish	½ fillet	½–1 fillet
Beans and lentils	2 tablespoons	3 tablespoons
Tofu/other soy products/Quorn	½–1 soy or quorn/grain burger, or 2 tablespoons ground meat	1 soy or quorn/grain burger, or 3 tablespoons ground meat
Eggs	1 egg	1–2 eggs
Nuts	Small handful	Small handful

Two portions a day can be achieved by eating

- a chicken or egg-salad sandwich (with minimal mayonnaise)
- a burrito made with ground beef, chicken, or tofu

ESSENTIAL FATS AND OILS

This group includes foods rich in essential fatty acids (the omega-3 and omega-6 fatty acids; see page 39), nuts (walnuts, cashews, almonds, pecans, brazil nuts, pine nuts, peanuts), seeds (sesame, pumpkin, sunflower), cold-pressed seed and nut oils (flax, pumpkin, walnut, sesame, and sunflower), and oily fish (sardines, mackerel, salmon, trout).

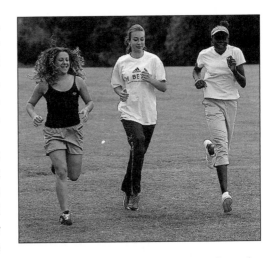

Peanut butter is a great source of these healthy oils, but read the label carefully before you buy! Most commercial brands contain added sugar and hydrogenated fats. Choose a brand that has no ingredients besides roasted, ground peanuts (and maybe some salt). You can even grind your own roasted peanuts into peanut butter at most natural-foods stores. Once a child develops a taste for this kind of peanut butter, the sugar-laden brands will seem unpalatable to them.

Choose plain, unsalted nuts and avoid those with coatings or flavorings. Lightly toast nuts and seeds under a grill or in a hot oven for a few minutes to bring out their wonderful nutty flavor.

Younger children may find certain nuts and seeds quite hard and may fail to chew them properly. In this case, ground nuts and seeds (ready-bought or ground in a coffee grinder at home) are most beneficial. Sprinkle them on salads, granola, or stews. You can even stir them into fruit smoothies.

The nutritional value of nuts, seeds, and oils is easily destroyed by heating and by exposure to light and air. Therefore, store them in dark bottles in a cool, dark place.

A typical child portion is:

	5–10 YEARS	11–15 YEARS
Nuts and seeds	1 tablespoon	1 heaping tablespoon
Nut and seed oils, peanut butter	1 teaspoon	1 tablespoon
Oily fish*	2 oz. fish	3 oz. fish

*Oily fish is the richest source of omega-3 oils; 1–2 servings a week would more than cover a child's needs.

Nut Allergies

Nut allergies seem to be appearing in young children more often than they used to. It is estimated that one in two hundred children may be allergic to peanuts. The exact cause is unknown, but children with nut allergies often have other allergies and other allergy-related conditions such as asthma, hay fever, and eczema. A family history of allergy also increases the risk of a child's developing a nut allergy. Early signs may include a mild tingling in the mouth or more obvious swelling in the mouth, difficulty breathing and swallowing, culminating, occasionally, in anaphylactic shock, which can kill if not dealt with quickly.

The current recommendation is that children under three years old with a personal or family history of allergy should not be given peanuts in any form. Children with no allergy history can be given peanuts and other nut products after the age of one. Whole nuts and crunchy nut butters should not be given to children under five years old because of the risk of choking.

One portion a day can be achieved by eating

- a small handful of nuts or seeds

  OR

- a tablespoon of oil added to a dressing or sauce

  OR

- a peanut butter sandwich

FATTY AND SUGARY FOODS

This group includes cookies, cakes, sweets, soft drinks, chocolate and other candy, and chips. Aim to limit these foods to once a day because they are high in saturated fat and/or added sugar. They supply relatively large numbers of calories with few, if any, essential nutrients (empty calories).

The major problem is that if your child eats a lot of these foods, she or he will have little room left for nutritious foods. Children can develop a taste for intensely sweet, salty processed foods, which takes them even farther away from the taste of more natural foods. In other words, sugary, fatty foods displace healthy foods from a child's diet. Of course, these foods should not be totally banned from a healthy diet. The idea is to eat them only in moderation, and to regard them as extras or treats.

Children will get all the fats they need from foods in the essential-oils group (nuts, seeds, oils, oily fish), dairy foods, and protein-rich foods. Added sugars are, strictly speaking, unnecessary, but can be used sparingly to enhance the flavor of healthy foods (for example, jam spread on whole-grain toast). Encourage your child to enjoy the more natural sweetness of fruit, natural fruit juice, dried fruit, and fruit desserts. Steer them away from artificially sweetened foods and intensely sugary foods, such as sweetened breakfast cereals and artificially flavored/colored fruit punch.

Looking after Children's Teeth

Eating lots of sugary foods increases the chances of tooth decay, but so do many other foods. Any carbohydrate-containing food that sticks to the teeth will encourage decay, especially if it is eaten frequently throughout the day. Acidic foods and drinks should also be avoided because they cause enamel erosion–literally dissolving the tooth away. There are a number of things you can encourage your children to do to prevent tooth decay and erosion:

- Brush their teeth with a little fluoride toothpaste, ideally after each meal. Aim for a minimum of twice a day, after breakfast and before bed.

- Avoid sweet or sugary foods and drinks between meals.

- Avoid sugary foods or drinks within an hour of bedtime–water or milk are the only "safe" drinks.

- Limit acidic drinks, such as soft drinks, fruit punch, and fruit juice, to mealtime.

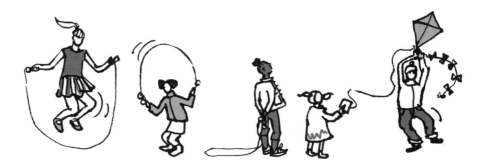

- Encourage water between meals, alternatively milk or very diluted fruit juice.

- Avoid sticky foods between meals, including candy, chocolate, cookies, raisins and other dried fruit, and fruit bars. These leave residues on the teeth, increasing the risk of decay. Note: dried fruit is as potentially harmful to teeth as sweets!

- If sugary foods or drinks are eaten, it is better to finish them quickly than it is to eat the sweets or sip the drink over an hour or more.

- Encourage the drinking of acidic drinks with a straw. This reduces the contact of the drink with the teeth. Sugar-free drinks are not necessarily better for children's teeth as they are quite acidic and can cause dental erosion.

- Have some cheese, plain yogurt, milk, or nuts at the end of a meal. These foods are "safe" for teeth. Eating cheese at the end of a meal or as a snack encourages remineralization of tooth enamel and so helps counteract the harmful effects of sugar and acids.

Snacks and Drinks That Are Safer for Teeth

SNACKS	DRINKS
Fresh fruit	Water
Yogurt (preferably unsweetened)	Milk
Cheese (with crackers or bread)	Diluted fruit juice (2 parts water to 1 part juice)
Toast, plain or with peanut butter (without added sugar) or cheese	
Nuts	
Crudités with dips	
Sandwiches	

CHAPTER 3

Protein Power

Children need protein to help them grow and develop properly. Protein also makes up your child's muscles, organs, skin, and hair. Some protein converts to fuel, supplying energy to exercising muscles. Does that mean active children need more protein? Will extra protein benefit children's performance and make them stronger? This chapter explains why protein is needed and how much protein children should eat. It gives you a guide to planning balanced meals containing the right amounts of protein. If your children do not eat meat, you need to be aware of the nutritional pitfalls. Here you'll find practical advice on vegetarian protein alternatives and how to plan a vegetarian diet.

What Happens to Protein in the Body?

When protein is eaten, it is broken down in the gut into its constituent amino acids. These are absorbed into the bloodstream, taken to the body's cells, and then reassembled into new proteins, where they may be used for

- building, maintaining, and repairing body cells and organs
- making hormones and enzymes, which regulate body functions
- making antibodies, which fight germs and illnesses

Children's bodily tissues and organs are by no means fixed; they are constantly being broken down and rebuilt. This process of repair and renewal

25

takes place much faster in children than in adults. That's why you need to make sure they get a regular supply of protein in their diet.

Will Extra Protein Make Stronger Muscles?

Muscles are made mainly out of protein and water. It's tempting, then, to think that extra protein will help children build bigger and stronger muscles. Or that it will make their muscles work better and improve their performance in sports. But it's not quite that simple.

In order to grow, your child's muscles need hormones called *androgens,* coupled with protein and regular exercise. Androgen levels rise during puberty in both boys and girls, accounting for their growth spurt. Boys have higher androgen levels than girls, so they tend to grow bigger muscles. But androgen won't do a good job on its own; children still need to get enough protein and to exercise regularly if they want strong muscles.

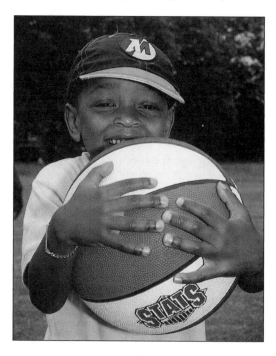

How Much Protein?

Because children are growing rapidly they need more protein relative to their weight than adults do. The recommended intakes for protein published by the U.S. Food and Nutrition Board establish general guidelines for boys and girls of different ages. These are given in the table below. Most children need about 1 gram (g) of protein per kilogram (kg) of body weight. (Adults need about 0.80 g/kg.) For example, a ten-year-old who weighs 40 kg should eat about 40 g of protein daily. (To determine body weight in kilograms, divide pounds by 2.2. For example, 75 pounds equals 34 kg.) However, the published values do not take exercise into account. Children who are very active or who train very hard may need a little more protein.

Daily Protein Requirements of Children[8]		
AGE GROUP	**BOYS**	**GIRLS**
4–8 years	19 g	19 g
9–13 years	34 g	34 g
14–18 years	52 g	46 g

How to Get Enough Protein

Active children can easily meet their protein needs with a daily diet that includes two portions from the Food Pyramid's protein-rich group (lean meat, fish, poultry, eggs, beans, lentils, nuts, and soy), as well as foods from the grain group (bread, rice, pasta, cereals) and dairy group (milk, yogurt, cheese), which also supply some protein. Encourage your children to eat a variety of foods from each group. The protein content of various foods is shown in the table on page 000. Getting enough protein is unlikely to be a problem if children include animal sources of protein on a daily basis (meat, poultry, fish, dairy foods, and eggs).

What about Vegetarian Diets?

To get enough protein from a vegetarian diet, children need to eat a wide variety of plant proteins (see box titled "Other Dietary Considerations for Vegetarians" on page 29). Doing so will ensure that they get the right combination of the amino acids essential for growth. There are nine essential amino acids (EAAs), so called because they must be supplied in the diet and cannot be made in the body. Since plant proteins (beans, lentils, soy, grains, nuts) contain smaller amounts of EAAs than animal proteins (meat, poultry, fish, eggs), you need to combine two or more of the plant foods to get the right balance of EAAs. Suitable combinations include:

- Red lentil marinara sauce and pasta
- Hummus (chickpea dip) and pita bread
- Vegetarian chili with rice
- Peanut butter sandwich
- Veggie burrito containing pinto beans (or black beans) with tortilla (wheat or corn)

Protein in Various Foods

FOOD	SERVING SIZE	PROTEIN (GRAMS)
Meat and fish		
Lean beef, grilled	1 slice (2 oz.)	15
Chicken breast, grilled	2 thin slices (2.25 oz.)	20
Cod, poached	1 small fillet (3 oz.)	18
Tuna, canned in water	½ can (1¾ oz.)	12
Dairy foods		
Cheese, cheddar	2 slices (1.5 oz.)	10
Skim milk	1 glass (8 fluid oz.)	7
Low-fat yogurt, fruit	1 carton (8 oz.)	6
Eggs	1 egg	8
Nuts and seeds		
Nuts and seeds (most varieties)	handful (1 oz.)	6
Peanut butter	1 tablespoon (¾ oz.)	5
Dried beans, legumes		
Baked beans	1 small can (8 oz.)	10
Red lentils, boiled	3 tablespoons (4 oz.)	9
Cooked beans, most varieties	3 tablespoons (4 oz.)	10
Soy products		
Tofu	2 tablespoons (1 oz.)	13
Veggie burger	1 burger (2 oz.)	5

- Black-eyed peas and cornbread
- Soy burger in a bun

Other Dietary Considerations for Vegetarians

A vegetarian diet can be perfectly sound as long as children eat a wide variety of foods from each of the groups in the Food Pyramid. Problems arise only when suitable foods are not substituted for meat. Besides protein, the nutrients most at risk are:

- Iron—obtain from whole-grain bread and cereal foods, green leafy vegetables (broccoli, spinach), beans, lentils, nuts, seeds, and iron-fortified breakfast cereals. Offer a vitamin C–rich food or drink (e.g., fruit or fruit juice) at mealtimes, as vitamin C increases iron absorption.
- Vitamin B-12—obtain from dairy foods, eggs, fortified breakfast cereals, and fortified soy products.
- Calcium—obtain from dairy foods, seeds, calcium-fortified soy products, almonds, and oranges.

Sometimes older children—mainly girls—adopt a vegetarian or vegan diet in a misguided attempt to lose weight. If they fail to substitute suitable foods for meat, or if they eat only a very limited range of foods, they may be at risk of developing a nutritional deficiency or an eating disorder. If you are concerned, seek advice from a registered dietitian, nutritionist, or eating-disorder specialist (see Chapter 12, "Eating Disorders").

What about Protein Supplements?

Protein supplements and meal-replacement products containing protein are unnecessary for children. Even the very active should be able to get enough protein from their diet. While such supplements may a have a role to play in the diets of some adult athletes, there is no justification for giving them to children. It is more important that children learn how to plan a balanced diet from ordinary foods and how to get protein from the right food combinations.

CHAPTER 4

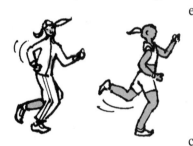

Carb-Charging

Although many popular diets today encourage adults to limit or cut out carbohydrates entirely, it is important to remember that carbohydrate foods are energy foods. Active children need plenty of them not only to fuel their activity but also to support their growth. But between eating too many sugary foods and too few grains and fruit, it's often difficult to get the balance of carbs in the diet right. Get it wrong and children may experience flagging energy levels and mood swings. This chapter explains how much carbohydrate kids should eat and helps you to plan a balanced daily diet. It considers which types of carbohydrates are best for health and how to combine different carbohydrates to ensure sustained energy throughout the day.

Why Do Kids Need Carbs?

The body turns carbohydrate into glucose, which is then circulated in the blood. Most of the glucose is not needed right away, so it is stored as glycogen in the liver and in the muscles. The main purpose of liver glycogen is to maintain steady blood-glucose levels, evening out any peaks and troughs, and keeping a steady supply to fuel the brain. Muscle glycogen, on the other hand, is used to provide fuel for the muscles to do work. Whenever children exercise, muscle glycogen is broken down to supply energy.

How Much Carbohydrate?

It is recommended that active children obtain around 50–60 percent of their calories from carbohydrate. For example, a child who requires two thousand calories per day would need to eat 250–300 grams of carbohydrate (there are four calories per gram of carbohydrate). A good guide is to give children six to eight portions (depending on their size and energy requirements) from the grain group in the Food Pyramid–bread, pasta, rice, noodles, breakfast cereals, oatmeal and other hot cereals, crackers, and starchy vegetables such as potatoes, sweet potatoes, parsnips, and yams–as well as two portions from the fruit group, and two to three portions from the dairy group, which also provide some carbohydrate. (See Chapter 2 for details about the Food Pyramid.) The exact portion size depends on your child's calorie needs. Generally, older, heavier, and more active children need bigger portions. Be guided by their appetite, but don't get too prescriptive about the exact amount they should eat. Check the carbohydrate content of various foods in the table on pages 34–36.

The following sample menu would be suitable for an active boy aged seven to ten years. It provides about two thousand calories. It supplies approximately 55 percent of calories from carbohydrate, 15–20 percent from protein, and 25–30 percent from fat.

Sample Menu for Boy 7–10 Years Old	
Breakfast	Oatmeal with raisins and a little honey Orange juice
Snack	Apple and mandarin orange, water
Lunch	Peanut butter or tuna sandwich on whole-grain bread Cut-up carrot and cucumber Yogurt, grapes Water or diluted fruit juice
Snack (before training)	Cereal bar or bananas, water
Snack (after training)	Dried fruit, water

Dinner	Marvelous Macaroni and Cheese (see
	  recipe on page 147), steamed broccoli,
	  and carrots
	Fruit cobbler, water

Which Types of Carbohydrate Are Best?

The best carbohydrate foods—whole-grain bread, whole-grain cereals, brown rice, pasta, beans, lentils, potatoes, sweet potatoes, fresh fruit, and dried fruit—supply more than just energy. They provide other important nutrients too—B vitamins, iron, zinc, magnesium, and fiber—needed for children's growth and development. Make sure that the majority of children's carbohydrate needs come from these unrefined foods.

Highly processed carbohydrate foods, such as white bread, cookies, sugar, sugary breakfast cereals, candy, pastries, and soft drinks, should be eaten far less often. The drawback with these foods is that most of the vital nutrients have been lost during processing. White bread, for example, contains much less fiber, iron, zinc, magnesium, and B vitamins than whole-grain bread. Sweets and sugar are virtually devoid of nutrients, providing mostly "empty calories," and so should be kept to a minimum.

The other downside of highly refined foods is that they are high-glycemic foods, or fast-releasing energy foods. This means they are converted into blood glucose rapidly. If children rely on lots of high-glycemic foods for energy, they may develop problems with blood-glucose control, a problem that can eventually lead to type-II diabetes. At the very least, you'll certainly notice a change in their energy levels and mood. Such a diet is certainly unsuitable for training and sports.

Let's consider what happens when children eat a couple of cookies or a chocolate bar. The sugars in these foods are broken down into glucose and absorbed very quickly, producing a rapid rise in blood-glucose levels. This

Fiber

Fiber offers three main benefits. First, it helps to keep children's digestive tracts healthy, allowing food to pass easily through the body and preventing constipation. Second, it helps slow the absorption of glucose into the blood, maintaining steady blood-glucose levels and energy levels. And that's vital for active children! Third, foods naturally rich in fiber (whole-grain bread, oatmeal, fruit, vegetables) are more filling and satisfying. Kids who've eaten a high-fiber meal won't get so hungry between meals and ask for sugary snacks.

Children can get all the fiber they need from whole-grain breads and cereals, fruit, vegetables, oats, brown rice, beans, lentils, and nuts. There's no need to add bran or lots of bran-enriched cereals.

signals to the pancreas to pump out extra insulin, which in turn causes blood-glucose levels to drop too quickly. This rapid downswing in blood glu-

cose can make many children feel tired, irritable, hungry, and unable to concentrate—a classic case of the "sugar blues"!

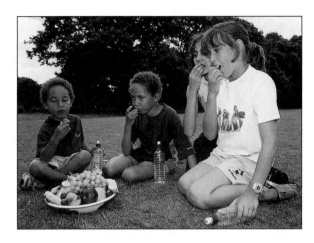

If you do give your child a high-glycemic food, it's a good idea to also include a protein-rich food (meat, poultry, fish, eggs, milk, cheese, or yogurt), a high-fat food (oil, butter, nuts, seeds), or a high-fiber food (fruit, vegetables, oats) in the same meal. These are low-glycemic foods (slow-releasing energy foods), which delay the absorption of glucose and so prevent the blood-glucose level from rising too rapidly and then falling fast.

Some examples of combinations of high-glycemic and low-glycemic foods are listed in the next section of this chapter.

Carbohydrates and the Glycemic Index

All types of carbohydrates are digested into simple sugars and then absorbed into the bloodstream. But eventually they all end up as glucose in the bloodstream. Some carbohydrate foods (the high-glycemic foods mentioned above) get there faster than others; this can make a big difference in children's energy levels and physical performance. That's why it's useful to know about the glycemic index (GI) of foods.

The GI of a carbohydrate food is an indication of how slowly or quickly it raises blood glucose levels. Glucose has a score of 100 because it enters the bloodstream faster than all other foods, giving a sharp rise in blood glucose. Foods that are more slowly digested and absorbed, such as potatoes, pasta, beans, and fruit, have a GI of less than 100 and cause a slower and more sustained rise in glucose levels. The GI of various foods is given in the table starting on the next page.

Glycemic Index (GI) and Carbohydrate Content of Selected Foods[9]

FOOD	PORTION SIZE	GI	CARBOHYDRATE (GRAMS)
Breakfast cereals			
Cornflakes	small bowl (30 g)	84	26
Rice Krispies	small bowl (30 g)	82	27
Cheerios	small bowl (30 g)	74	23
Shredded wheat	2 biscuits (45 g)	67	31
Weetabix	2 biscuits (40 g)	69	30
Oatmeal (made with water)	small bowl (160 g)	42	14
Granola	small bowl (50 g)	56	34
Grains/pasta			
Rice—brown	6 tbsp. (180 g)	76	58
Rice—white	6 tbsp. (180 g)	87	56
Rice—basmati	4 tbsp. (60 g)	58	48
Noodles—instant	4 tbsp. (230 g cooked)	46	30
Pasta, macaroni	4 tbsp. (230 g cooked)	45	43
Spaghetti	4 tbsp. (220 g cooked)	41	49
Bread			
White bread	1 large slice (36 g)	70	18
Whole-grain bread	1 large slice (38 g)	69	16
Pizza	1 large slice (115 g)	60	38
Crackers			
Rice cakes	1 (8 g)	85	6
Cookies and cakes			
Graham cracker	1 (15 g)	59	10
Shortbread	1 (13 g)	64	8
Oatmeal	1 (13 g)	55	8
Muffin	1 (68 g)	44	34
Sponge cake	1 slice (60 g)	46	39
Vegetables			
Parsnip	2 tbsp. (65 g)	97	8
Potato—baked	1 average (180 g)	85	22
Potato—boiled, new	7 small (175 g)	62	27
Potato—mashed	4 tbsp. (180 g)	70	28

Glycemic Index (GI) and Carbohydrate Content of Selected Foods (cont'd.)

FOOD	PORTION SIZE	GI	CARBOHYDRATE (GRAMS)
Carrots	2 tbsp. (60 g)	49	3
Peas	2 tbsp. (70 g)	48	7
Corn	2 tbsp. (85 g)	55	17
Sweet potato	1 medium (130 g)	54	27
Fries	average portion (165 g)	75	59
Legumes			
Baked beans	1 small can (205 g)	48	31
Chickpeas	4 tbsp. (140 g)	33	24
Red kidney beans	4 tbsp. (120 g)	27	20
Lentils (red)	4 tbsp. (160 g)	26	28
Fruit			
Pineapple	1 slice (80 g)	66	8
Raisins	1 tbsp. (30 g)	64	21
Apricot	1 (40 g)	57	3
Banana	1 (100 g)	55	23
Grapes	small bunch (100 g)	46	15
Kiwi fruit	1 (68 g)	52	6
Mango	½ (75 g)	55	11
Orange	1 (208 g)	44	12
Peach	1 (121 g)	42	8
Apple	1 (100 g)	38	12
Apricot (dried)	5 (40 g)	31	15
Cherries	small handful (100 g)	22	10
Pear	1 (160 g)	38	16
Plum	1 (55 g)	39	5
Beverages			
Apple juice	1 glass (160 ml)	40	16
Orange juice	1 glass (160 ml)	46	14
Snacks			
Tortilla chips	1 bag (50 g)	72	30
Potato chips	1 small bag (30 g)	54	16
Peanuts	small handful (50 g)	14	4
Dairy products			
Ice cream	1 scoop (60 g)	61	14

Glycemic Index (GI) and Carbohydrate Content of Selected Foods (cont'd.)

FOOD	PORTION SIZE	GI	CARBOHYDRATE (GRAMS)
Milk—whole	1 cup (300 ml)	27	14
Milk—skim	1 cup (300 ml)	32	15
Yogurt, fruit (low-fat)	1 carton (150 g)	33	27
Candy			
Mars bar	1 standard (65 g)	68	43
Granola bar	1 (33 g)	61	20
Milk chocolate	1 bar (54 g)	49	31
Sugars			
Glucose	1 tsp. (5 g)	100	5
Honey	1 heaping tsp. (17 g)	58	13
Sucrose (table sugar)	1 tsp. (5 g)	65	5

The closer the GI to 100, the faster the food is absorbed and turned into blood glucose. Sometimes—for example, after training—a high-GI snack is beneficial (see Chapter 7). But for the most part, eating lots of high-GI snacks is not a good idea, as they will leave children feeling lethargic.

Give children mostly low-GI meals and snacks. These are best because they provide long-lasting energy. Of course, kids don't need to eat only low-GI carbohydrates. By combining a high-GI carbohydrate with protein, fat, or another carbohydrate with a low GI, you automatically lower the overall GI of the meal. Here are some examples of simple meals that combine a high-GI carbohydrate with a low-GI food, resulting in an overall lower GI:

- Baked potato with cheese
- Tuna sandwich
- Cookie with an apple
- Toast with peanut butter
- Rice cakes with peanut butter
- Pasta with chicken
- Hummus on a bagel
- Cornflakes with milk
- Cake and yogurt

CHAPTER 5

Fat Matters

Fat is an important nutrient for children. It not only contributes to their caloric needs (i.e., provides energy), but certain types of fats are crucial for their growth and development. This chapter explains which fats are best for children and which ones should be avoided. You'll find a practical guide to the different types of fats and oils to help you untangle the jargon on food labels. Should children restrict their fat intake in order to avoid heart disease? Or will doing so put them at risk of malnutrition? This chapter tells you how much fat children should eat and offers some easy ways to cut down on unwanted fats.

Why Is Fat Needed?

Here are the main reasons why children need fat in their diet.

FOR FUEL

Fat supplies energy (calories) that can either be used immediately or stored for future use. In fact, children's fat stores play an important part in fuelling the muscles during many types of physical activity. For example, it takes oxygen, fat, and carbohydrates to create the extra energy needed to do certain aerobic activities, such as playing football, running in the playground, and swimming (see Chapter 7, "Eating for Action").

In addition, fat is used to make energy virtually all the time, even while sitting or walking. (The only exceptions are during all-out exercise such as sprinting, jumping, or throwing.) Since fat is a very concentrated source of energy (providing nine calories per gram, compared with four calories per gram for both carbohydrate and protein), it can be useful for meeting the energy needs of children who find it difficult to eat enough. On the other hand, those with larger appetites need to avoid consuming too much fat. Fatty foods such as chips, cookies, and chocolate are easy to overeat as they have little filling power. Guidelines for fat consumption appear later in the chapter.

FOR ABSORBING AND USING VITAMINS

Fat in food helps children's bodies absorb the fat-soluble vitamins A, D, E, and K. A fat-free meal (e.g., baked potato, carrots, and peas) would render any fat-soluble vitamins useless. By contrast, including a small amount of fat or oil in the meal (e.g., adding margarine or cheese to the potato) helps the body absorb the vitamin A in the carrots. Fats also transport nutrients, such as vitamins and proteins, around the body.

FOR GROWTH, DEVELOPMENT, AND PEAK HEALTH

Certain kinds of fats and oils are needed for normal growth and development. These are the unsaturated fats, in particular the essential fats (see below). Fats are also an important part of the membranes of all body cells. Without fat, cells simply couldn't exist. But to function at their best, cells need the right ratio of different fats.

FOR TASTE AND TEXTURE

Fat contributes to the taste and the texture of many foods and so makes eating more enjoyable. With too little fat, many foods become unpalatable. Too much, of course, can be harmful. It's a question of balance.

What's the Difference Between Saturated and Unsaturated Fats?

In simple terms, saturated fats are solid at room temperature, whereas unsaturated fats are liquid. Saturated fats generally come from animal products. For example, the fat in dairy foods and meat is high in saturated fats. However, there are two exceptions: coconut oil and palm (or palm kernel) oil. Despite being vegetable fats, they are both highly saturated. You'll find them in lots of processed foods, such as cookies, margarine, cakes, desserts, snack bars, and pies. If the label simply says "vegetable fat," chances are it's made from coconut or palm oil. Try to keep saturated fats to a minimum (see guidelines below) because they raise levels of cholesterol in the blood—both in children and adults. There is, in fact, no actual need for saturated fats in the diet!

Unsaturated fats generally come from plants. There are two types of unsaturated fats: monounsaturated and polyunsaturated. Monounsaturated fats are found in olives, olive oil, canola (rapeseed) oil, avocados, nuts and their oils, and seeds and their oils. Polyunsaturated fats are found in sunflower, corn, and other vegetable oils, and in oily fish. Both monounsaturated and polyunsaturated fats lower the level of "bad" cholesterol in the blood, so they help to reduce the risk of heart disease in later life. But monounsaturated fats offer additional health benefits. Unlike polyunsaturated fats, they maintain levels of "good" cholesterol in the blood while lowering levels of "bad" cholesterol.

What Are the Essential Fats?

The essential fatty acids (EFAs) are vital for both children's and adults' health. They cannot be made in the body so they must be supplied in the diet. There are two families of EFAs, the omega-3 oils and the omega-6 oils. Oily fish (sardines, salmon, mackerel), pumpkin seeds, walnuts, green leafy vegetables, soybeans, omega-3 enriched eggs, sweet potatoes, and certain oils (flaxseed, pumpkin seed, walnut, soy, and canola) are the best sources of omega-3s. Most other vegetable oils (e.g., sunflower, safflower, corn), nuts, seeds, and whole grains are rich in omega-6s. We need both to be healthy, but most of us get too few omega-3s in relation to omega-6s. It's especially important for children to get enough omega-3s. They need them for brain growth and development. These oils also help to lower blood fats and to improve oxygen delivery to all body cells. And because omega-3s enhance aerobic metabolism, a diet rich in them will help children's sports performance.

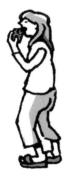

What Is Hydrogenated Fat?

Hydrogenated fat is made from vegetable oil that has been hardened or hydrogenated. In this process hydrogen is added to the oil to saturate the fatty-acid molecules so that it effectively becomes a saturated fat. This new fat is solid at room temperature, rather like butter or lard. Food manufacturers like hydrogenated fat because it is cheap, tasteless, and less likely to become rancid than other fats. You'll find it in literally thousands of products: cakes, cookies, pies, pastries, snack bars, cereal bars, crackers, puddings, ice cream, and chocolate candy.

The big problem with hydrogenated fat, apart from being highly saturated, is that it also contains trans fats. These are formed during the hydro-

Sources of Fat		
TYPE OF FAT	**FOUND IN**	**GOOD OR BAD?**
Saturated	Meat, burgers, sausages, butter, whole milk, cheese, cream, products containing palm or coconut oil ("vegetable fat"), some margarines.	Bad. It raises blood cholesterol and increases heart disease and cancer risk.
Hydrogenated	Margarine, cookies, bars, cakes, pies, pastries, other bakery goods.	Bad. Contains trans fats, which increase heart disease and cancer risk.
Polyunsaturated	Vegetable oils (e.g., sunflower, corn), vegetable-oil margarine, oily fish, nuts.	Good. Lowers "bad" cholesterol levels.
Omega-6	Vegetable oils (e.g., sunflower, corn), vegetable-oil margarine, nuts, seeds.	Good. Essential for health.
Omega-3	Oily fish, walnuts, pumpkin seeds, soybeans, omega-3 enriched eggs, sweet potatoes.	Excellent. Essential for overall health and brain development, lowers risk of heart attacks and stroke in adulthood, improves sports performance.
Monounsaturated	Olive oil, olives, avocados, nuts, seeds, canola (rapeseed) oil.	Good. Lowers "bad" cholesterol, maintains "good" cholesterol levels. Reduces heart disease and cancer risk.

genation process as some of the fat molecules change shape. Trans fats are harmful because they raise "bad" cholesterol levels and lower "good" cholesterol levels: a double whammy for increasing heart-disease risk.

Trans fats are not listed as such on food labels. The only way to avoid them is to check food labels for the words "hydrogenated fat" or "partially hydrogenated fat" (or, sometimes, "hydrogenated vegetable oil" or "partially hydrogenated vegetable oil"). It's worrisome to consider how many foods specifically targeted to children contain these hydrogenated fats. Be warned.

How Much Fat Should Children Eat?

Getting the balance right is the key. Removing too much fat from children's diets can be harmful because it may result in their failing to get enough calories, fat-soluble vitamins, and essential fats, and their growth and development may suffer. Children need slightly more fat relative to their weight and calorie intake compared with adults. It's important that they get enough calories not only to fuel physical activity but also to support growth.

On the other hand, too much fat will result in excess body fat, reduced physical performance, and all the associated risks of obesity (see Chapter 9, "Overweight Kids"). The table below gives the fat content of various foods.

Children aged five to fifteen years should get between 25 percent and 35 percent of calories from fat. For example, a ten-year-old boy who eats two

Fat Content of Selected Foods	
FOOD	**FAT CONTENT**
Plain hamburger (110 g)	10 g
Fries (average portion, 110 g)	17 g
2 chocolate cookies	8 g
1 chocolate candy bar	12 g
1 bag (30 g) of potato chips	10 g
1 chocolate-coated cereal bar (24 g)	7 g
2 sausages (20 g each)	8 g
1 cupcake (30 g)	4 g

thousand calories a day should get between fifty-five and seventy-eight grams of fat (there are nine calories in one gram of fat). The majority of this should come from "good" fats—that is, the unsaturated fats. As a guide, include at least one portion daily from the essential fats group of the Food Pyramid (nuts, seeds, seed and nut oils, and oily fish—see Chapter 2). Foods from the protein-rich group and dairy group will also supply some fat.

Less than 10 percent of daily calories should come from saturated fats. The Food Pyramid recommends eating no more than one portion per day from the sugary and fatty foods group.

Ten Easy Ways to Reduce Fat (Without Missing Out on Essential Nutrients)

1. Serve smaller portions of meat, and choose leaner varieties. Trim off any visible fat.

2. Use full-fat dairy products in moderation. Swap whole milk for low-fat or skim milk.

3. Reduce consumption of processed and fatty meat products (sausages, cold cuts, burgers).

4. Limit fast food (don't serve these daily): burgers, pizza with fatty meat toppings, nuggets, fried chicken, hot dogs, fries.

5. Limit high-fat snack foods: chocolate bars, cookies, chips, muffins, doughnuts, croissants.

6. Serve lower-fat desserts (e.g., yogurt, frozen yogurt, fresh fruit) in place of high-fat ones.

7. Keep pastries and pies to a minimum.

8. Provide homemade, lower-fat muffins, cakes, cookies, scones, bagels, and English muffins in place of traditional or store-bought cakes and cookies (see recipes in Chapter 20, "Kids' Snacks").

9. Offer fresh fruit, dried fruit, rice cakes, or fruit bars in place of cookies.

10. Serve baked potatoes or homemade Oven Potato Wedges (see recipe on page 182) in place of fries and chips.

CHAPTER 6

Vitamins and Minerals

Vitamins and minerals are substances that are needed in tiny amounts to enable your child's body to work properly and prevent illness.

What Do Vitamins and Minerals Do?

There are thirteen different vitamins, which support almost every system in the body, including the immune system and the brain and nervous system. Many of them help to convert food into energy and help the body to use carbohydrate, fat, and protein. They are also involved in regulating growth, making red blood cells, and protecting the body against harmful free radicals.

The fifteen minerals have mainly structural roles (such as depositing calcium in the teeth and bones) or regulatory roles (such as controlling fluid balance and muscle contraction). Iron is one of the most important minerals for active children as it is essential for the production of hemoglobin (the oxygen-carrying pigment in red blood cells). The section titled "Guide to Vitamins and Minerals," below, tells you more about the functions and food sources of the key vitamins and minerals.

How to Get Enough Vitamins and Minerals

Your children should be able to meet their vitamin and mineral needs by eating the recommended number of portions from each food group in the

What Are Daily Values, RDAs, and DRIs?

You will find the term "% Daily Value" on food and supplement labels. These "Daily Values" are rough estimates of nutrient requirements judged by a group of experts to cover the needs of most people. If, for example, a label says "Calcium 2%," that means one serving of the product in question supplies 2 percent of the calcium needed each day by an average person on a two-thousand-calorie diet. Where do these "Daily Values" come from? In the United States, the Food and Nutrition Board, part of the federal agency known as the Institute of Medicine, has established Recommended Daily Amounts (RDAs) (or, strictly speaking, Dietary Reference Intakes, DRIs) for boys and girls in different age categories. (DRIs are also established for adults in different life stages.) The "Daily Values" referred to on food labels are based on an averaging of the various DRIs.

DRIs are designed to prevent deficiency symptoms, allow for a little storage of the nutrient, and cover differences in need from one individual to the next. They are not targets; rather they are guidelines to help you make sure that your child is getting enough nutrients. If you think your child is regularly eating less than the DRIs, you should see a qualified nutritionist or see a dietitian.

Food Pyramid (Chapter 2). They should aim for two portions from the fruit group, three portions from the vegetable group, two to three portions from the dairy group, two portions from the protein-rich group, six to eight portions from the grains group, and one portion from the essential fats group. Vary the choices of foods from each group as much as possible.

How Can You Get Children to Eat More Fruits and Vegetables?

It is often a struggle to get children to eat the recommended five daily portions of fruits and vegetables. National surveys in Great Britain have revealed that, on average, children eat fewer than two portions a day, a third of the recommended amount! Studies of U.S. kids show similarly dismal patterns. This means that many children are almost certainly missing out on important vitamins and minerals. Here are some ideas for encouraging them to eat more fruits and vegetables:

- Let children plant and harvest their own vegetable garden.
- Get children involved with the shopping. Let them choose (and, hopefully, eat) a new variety of fruits and vegetables.

- Get children involved with washing, peeling, and cutting vegetables.

- Aim to include two different vegetables with the main meal (usually dinner) and at least one vegetable with lunch. Mix colors.

- Aim to include two different fruits, either as snacks or at mealtimes (see the following suggestions).

- Establish healthy snack habits, making fresh fruit (whole or cut into bite-sized pieces), carrot, cucumber, and pepper matchsticks the norm for at least one snack daily.

- Set a good example yourself. Children are more likely to eat fruits and vegetables if they see you enjoying these foods daily and if there is a plentiful supply in the house.

- Children are more likely to eat small portions of two or three different vegetables than one large portion.

- Top breakfast cereal or yogurt with chopped fruit, e.g., strawberries, bananas, grated apple.

- Crudités (perhaps served with hummus, salsa, or a cheese dip) make good lunchbox foods (see Chapter 11, "Eating at School").

- Think outside the "meat and two veggies" box. All-in-one meals transform vegetables into dishes in their own right: think vegetable stew, vegetable stir-fry, and vegetable chili.

- Instead of tuna or cheese in baked potatoes, try steamed veggies or corn.

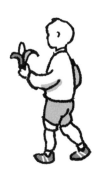

- The tomato in pasta sauce counts as a portion, but next time, throw in a cupful of chopped broccoli, peppers, zucchini, or mushrooms.

- Pass the fruit bowl around after dinner.

- Fruit smoothies and shakes are a delicious way to get a portion or two of fruit. Purée strawberries and banana with orange juice and ice cubes.

- Hide vegetables (e.g., carrots, mushrooms, spinach) in marinara sauce, soups, lasagnas, stews, bakes, and pies.

- Include lettuce and tomatoes in sandwiches, or serve them on the side.

- For younger children, make vegetables more fun. Arrange broccoli

Organic Food

Is organic food better for children? Should you consider switching to an organic diet for the whole family? According to a 2001 report from the Soil Association, in Great Britain, organic food is most definitely healthier, as well as safer.

Perhaps the only drawback to organic food is its higher cost. If you can afford it, incorporating even a few organic ingredients will be a step in the right direction. If you can't buy many organic foods, don't worry. It's important that your child eat plentiful amounts of fresh foods—even if they are nonorganic—rather than skimp on quantities.

Here are four reasons for going organic:

1. Organic foods contain the lowest possible amounts of contaminants such as pesticides, antibiotics, and nitrates. Although it remains a controversial issue, there is evidence that the "cocktail" effect of pesticide residues over time may cause health problems in the future.

2. Organic foods may have higher vitamin-C levels (the nutrient most easily destroyed), and higher levels of minerals such as calcium, iron, potassium, zinc, and magnesium.

3. Organic foods undergo minimal processing. That means they contain no hydrogenated fats, artificial additives, preservatives, or genetically modified organisms (GMOs).

4. Many organic foods taste better and have more flavor.

Going Organic

Here are some pointers for including more organic foods in your family's diet:

- Buy fruits and vegetables in season, when they are cheaper.

- Identify your family's six most frequently eaten foods and try to find organic equivalents.

- Start with lettuces, fruits, and vegetables. Of all the food groups, these have the highest pesticide residues; buying organic is the best way to avoid them.

- Join a local produce co-op, or visit a farmer's market—they offer the best values on organic produce.

- Snap up seasonal offers or promotions.

and cauliflower as trees on a base of mashed potato; or make faces (e.g., use carrots for eyes, baby corn for a nose, red peppers for the mouth, broccoli for hair, or whatever else your child likes).

- Let children decorate their own pizzas with a selection of peppers, mushrooms, tomatoes, and pineapple.

- Instead of sticking to the same vegetables prepared the same way, try new combinations and cooking techniques, e.g., cut carrots, parsnips, turnips, zucchini, and peppers into chunks, toss in a little olive oil, and bake in the oven.

- Add plenty of vegetables to soups (purée or leave chunky), curries, and stews.

- Enliven steamed vegetables with a little grated cheese.

- Younger children who refuse most vegetables will often eat "finger" vegetables, such as sugar-snap peas, baby corn, green beans, baby carrots, and cherry tomatoes.

- Add a few spoonfuls of frozen peas, corn, or canned kidney beans to the saucepan while cooking pasta or rice.

- Fruit cut into bite-sized pieces may be more attractive than whole fruit for younger children.

- Children can easily get bored with the same fruit (such as apples and bananas). Try exotic fruit (such as mangoes or pineapples) or berries (such as strawberries or blueberries) at least once a week.

- Use fruit in desserts. Try baked apples and bananas, fruit mixed with yogurt, rice pudding topped with fruit, fruit crumbles. See the recipes on pages 184–192.

Guide to Vitamins and Minerals

This section explains what the various vitamin and minerals do and how much a ten-year-old boy or girl needs to eat to achieve the RDA. Obviously, requirements vary with age, so younger children will usually need slightly less, older children slightly more. (Note: µg = micrograms; mg = milligrams.)

VITAMIN A is needed for growth, healthy eyesight, healthy skin, and for color and night vision.

Where to Get It: Full-fat dairy products, meat, liver, egg yolk, oily fish, margarine, butter. It can also be made in the body from beta-carotene (see below).

How Much? Get the RDA (600 µg) for vitamin A from a slice (40 g) of liver, or a glass (8 fluid oz.) of full-fat milk, plus two tablespoons (30 g) of margarine and one egg.

BETA-CAROTENE is an antioxidant. Antioxidants trap and destroy the free radicals that can damage cells and increase cancer risk (see the section titled "Antioxidants" in Chapter 6). The body also converts beta-carotene into vitamin A.

Where to Get It: Fruits and vegetables, especially orange, red, and yellow ones, e.g., carrots, apricots, peppers, tomatoes, mangoes, broccoli, winter squash, cantaloupe, pumpkin.

How Much? There is no official RDA, but you can get the suggested amount (15 mg) from two carrots, half a red pepper, and a slice of cantaloupe.

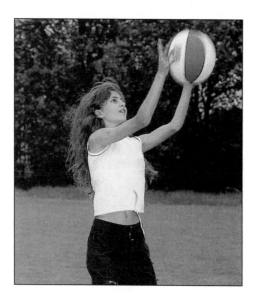

VITAMIN B-1 (THIAMIN) releases energy from carbohydrates. It is also needed for a healthy nervous system and digestive system.

Where to Get It: Whole-grain breads and cereals, beans, lentils, nuts, meat, sunflower seeds.

How Much? Get the RDA (0.9 mg) from three slices of whole-grain bread and a small handful of brazil nuts or peanuts.

VITAMIN B-2 (RIBOFLAVIN) releases energy from carbohydrates. It is also vital for healthy skin, eyes, and nerves.

Where to Get It: Milk and dairy products, meat, eggs, soy products.

How Much? Get the RDA (0.9 mg) from a small bowl of fortified breakfast cereal, a glass of milk, and a container of yogurt.

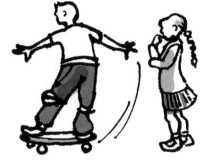

VITAMIN B-3 (NIACIN) releases energy from carbohydrates. It also promotes healthy skin, nerves, and digestion.

Where to Get It: Meat, nuts, milk and dairy products, eggs, whole-grain cereals.

How Much? Get the RDA (12 mg) from two slices of chicken, two slices of whole-grain bread, and one egg.

VITAMIN B-6 (PYRIDOXINE) helps the body to use protein, carbohydrate, and fat properly. It is essential for manufacturing red blood cells and for keeping the immune system working well.

Where to Get It: Beans, lentils, nuts, eggs, cereals, fish, bananas.

How Much? Get the RDA (1.0 mg) from a banana, a portion of white fish, and a peanut butter sandwich.

FOLIC ACID is needed for the formation of DNA and of the hemoglobin in red blood cells. It protects against heart disease in later life. It is especially essential for pregnant women to consume enough folic acid in order to ensure proper development of the neural tube in the fetus.

Where to Get It: Green leafy vegetables, brewer's yeast, beans, lentils, nuts, legumes, citrus fruit.

How Much? Get the RDA (300 μg) from a bowl of fortified breakfast cereal, a portion of brussels sprouts, and a glass (8 fluid oz.) of orange juice. (The RDA for pregnant women is 600 μg.)

VITAMIN B-12 is essential for growth and for formation of red blood cells.

Where to Get It: Milk and dairy products, meat, fish, fortified breakfast cereals, soy products, and brewer's yeast.

How Much? Get the RDA (1.8 µg) from one egg, or two thin slices of red meat, or two bowls of fortified breakfast cereal.

VITAMIN C is a powerful antioxidant that protects cells from free-radical damage. It is also needed for the formation of healthy connective tissue, bones, teeth, blood vessels, gums, and teeth; it boosts immune function and helps iron absorption.

Where to Get It: Fruits and vegetables, especially raspberries, cantaloupe, kiwi fruit, oranges, grapefruit, strawberries, peppers, broccoli, cabbage, tomatoes.

How Much? Get the RDA (45 mg) from one kiwi fruit, or a small glass of orange juice, or two florets of broccoli.

VITAMIN D builds strong bones and teeth. It is needed to absorb calcium and phosphorus.

Where to Get It: Sunlight (the major source), oily fish, fortified milk, margarine, and breakfast cereals, eggs.

How Much? The RDA (5 µg) is based on the absence of adequate exposure to sunlight. Get it from a glass (8 fluid oz.) of fortified whole milk or one egg yolk.

VITAMIN E is an antioxidant. Antioxidants help to protect all cells from free radicals. Vitamin E also helps to prevent heart disease and promotes normal cell growth and development.

Where to Get It: Vegetable oils, oily fish, nuts, seeds, egg yolk, avocado.

How Much? Get the RDA (11 mg) from two tablespoons of hulled sunflower seeds, or a handful of (about twenty) almonds, or eight florets of broccoli with a slice of whole-grain toast and margarine.

CALCIUM is vital for building strong bones and teeth. It also helps with blood clotting and nerve and muscle function.

Where to Get It: Milk and dairy products, sardines, dark green leafy vegetables, beans, lentils, brazil nuts, almonds, figs, and sesame seeds.

How Much? Get the RDA (1,300 mg) from two glasses (8 fluid oz. each) of milk, a container of yogurt, and a thick slice of cheese.

Do Active Children Need More Calcium?

Calcium is a particularly important mineral for growing, active children. Along with phosphorus and magnesium it makes up the dense inner part of bones. It's important that children get plenty of calcium in their diet now because their bones are growing rapidly in length, width, and density. If their diet is low in calcium, some calcium will be taken out of the bones to keep the muscles and nerves functioning properly. This leaves the bones short-changed on calcium, putting them at risk of stress fractures and osteoporosis in later life. Around 90 percent of the maximum amount of bone mineral is achieved by the mid-teens, so now is the critical time for building up a good store in kids' bones.

But it's girls who are the biggest cause for concern with regard to calcium intake. A national survey of the dietary habits of American children found that fewer than 15 percent of girls ages eleven and over consumed the recommended number of servings of dairy foods, the richest source of calcium. Many adolescent girls shun dairy products in the mistaken belief that these foods are "fattening." Milk, for example, is substituted with soft drinks, and cheese is also avoided as fattening. While it can be a challenge to influence teenage girls' attitudes toward food, here are some ways of encouraging older children to meet their calcium requirements:

- Provide low-fat versions of dairy foods, such as skim and low-fat milk, low-fat yogurt, yogurt drinks, milkshakes or smoothies made with skim milk, and low-fat cheeses, including low-fat cottage cheese. Since teenagers tend to drink less plain milk, encourage them to eat more yogurt and yogurt drinks. Or try whipping up a smoothie made from calcium-fortified soy milk, or serving calcium-fortified soy milk with breakfast cereal. Explain that these are good ways of getting calcium.

- Discourage kids from consuming lots of soft drinks. Offer milkshakes made from skim milk or low-fat yogurt drinks instead.

- Provide other calcium-rich foods such as canned sardines and salmon (and other canned fish with edible bones), broccoli and other green leafy veggies, oranges, figs, tofu, and almonds.

- Talk to them about the importance of calcium and the risk of brittle bones.

- Be a good role model; consume calcium-rich foods yourself.

The two tables below give the daily calcium requirements for children of different ages and the amounts of various foods providing 200 mg of calcium, roughly one-fourth to one-sixth of the RDA.

DAILY CALCIUM REQUIREMENTS (MILLIGRAMS)		FOODS CONTAINING 200 MG CALCIUM	
4–8 years (boys and girls)	800	Milk	1 glass (⅔ cup)
9–18 years (boys and girls)	1,300	Milkshake	1 glass (⅔ cup)
		Cheddar cheese	1 slice (1 oz.)
		Yogurt	1 carton (6 oz.)
		Broccoli	10 sprigs (500 g)
		Oranges	3 oranges
		Sesame seeds	2 tbsp. (30 g)
		Tinned sardines	1½ (36 g)
		Almonds	50 nuts (83 g)
		Dried figs	4 figs (80 g)
		Pizza, cheese	1 slice (105 g)
		Tofu	1 slice (4 oz.)
		Ice cream	2½ scoops (250 g)

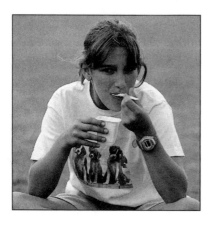

IRON is essential for the formation of hemoglobin (the oxygen-carrying pigment) in red blood cells. It is also needed for keeping the immune system working well, producing energy, and preventing anemia. Once girls start menstruating, their need for iron increases dramatically due to the monthly loss of blood.

Where to Get It: Meat, organ meat, whole-grain cereals, fortified breakfast cereals, beans, lentils, green leafy vegetables, nuts, sesame seeds, pumpkin seeds.

How Much? Get the RDA (8 mg) from one portion of beef chili or a bowl of fortified cereal, plus two portions of green leafy vegetables. (The RDA for menstruating girls increases to 15 mg, and it goes even higher after age eighteen.)

Do Active Children Need Extra Iron?

Because children and teenagers are growing, their need for iron is high. The requirement increases sharply during puberty when children have their growth spurt and when girls start menstruating. Iron is, of course, critical not only to good health but also for physical performance. Iron deficiency causes anemia, which limits oxygen transport in the blood and impairs physical performance.

But low iron stores—even without anemia—can cause chronic tiredness, lowered resistance to infection, loss of motivation, reduced mental performance, and disturbance of normal energy production in the muscles. For these reasons, getting enough iron in the diet is crucial for children. However, if you suspect that your child may be anemic or may even just suffer from iron deficiency, consult your doctor for a proper diagnosis before giving her or him iron supplements.

Studies looking at the diets of active children have found that many older girls and teenagers fail to reach the minimum iron requirement, putting them at risk of anemia. This may be due to their cutting down on red meat (a rich source of iron), coupled with the increased iron losses that occur during menstruation. If adolescent girls consume little red meat, they need to eat alternative iron sources, such as green leafy vegetables, whole-grain cereals, and beans. The absorption of iron is increased by consuming a vitamin C–rich food or drink at the same meal. For example, top a breakfast cereal with fruit, add broccoli to a pasta dish, have a glass of orange juice with lunch.

The tables below list the daily iron requirements for children and teenagers, and food portions providing 2 mg of iron, roughly one-fourth of the RDA for a ten-year-old.

DAILY IRON REQUIREMENT (MILLIGRAMS)		FOODS CONTAINING 2 MG IRON	
4–8 years (boys and girls)	10	Liver	½ thin slice (½ oz.)
9–13 years (boys and girls)	8	Beef	2 slices (87 g/3 oz.)
14–18 years (boys)	11	Baked beans	2 tbsp. (141 g)
14–18 years (girls)	15	Eggs	2 eggs
		Broccoli	4 florets (180 g)
		Cashew nuts	1 handful (33 g)
		Whole-grain bread	2 slices (40 g)
		Dried apricots	5 apricots (57 g)
		Lentils	2 tbsp. (80 g)

ZINC is needed for growth and cell repair. It helps wounds heal quickly and is an essential part of more than one hundred enzymes and hormones. It also keeps the immune system healthy and can help protect against colds.

Where to Get It: Eggs, whole-grain cereals, meat, nuts, and seeds.

How Much? Get the RDA (8 mg) from a portion of red meat and a handful of nuts or pumpkin seeds.

MAGNESIUM works with calcium to make healthy bones. It also assists in muscle and nerve function, regulating the beating of the heart, and the formation of healthy cells.

Where to Get It: Whole-grain cereals, fruits, vegetables, milk, nuts, and seeds.

How Much? Get the RDA (240 mg) from a small handful of almonds and three slices of whole-grain bread.

Do Active Children Need More Vitamins and Minerals?

Active children will need greater amounts of most vitamins and minerals compared to those who don't play sports. That's because regular exercise increases the demand for all the nutrients involved in energy production, cell repair, muscle function, and red-blood-cell formation. In particular, they will need higher amounts of the B vitamins (which help convert carbohydrate into energy), vitamins C and E (both antioxidants, which protect against the increased number of free radicals produced during exercise), and iron (needed to make extra hemoglobin to carry oxygen throughout the body).

If active children eat extra food to meet their increased caloric needs, then, providing they eat the right kinds of food, they should automatically be getting more vitamins and minerals.

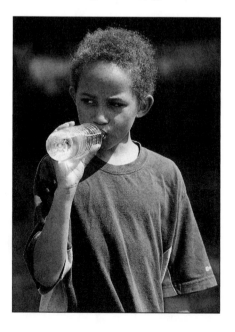

Should Children Take Vitamin Supplements?

In theory, children should not need supplements if they are eating a well-balanced diet and a wide variety of foods. But, in practice, few children

Keep the Vitamins In!

- Buy locally grown produce if you can, ideally from farmer's markets and local shops.

- If you can't buy local, at least buy American whenever possible. Imported produce is usually harvested while underripe (before it has developed its full vitamin quota) and will have lost much of its nutritional value during its journey to your supermarket.

- Buy fresh-looking, unblemished, undamaged fruits and vegetables.

- Do not buy fresh produce that is nearing its sell-by date.

- Do not buy ready-cut vegetables, salads, or fruit. They will have lost most of their nutritional value by the time you eat them.

- Prepare fruits and vegetables just before you make them into a salad or cook them. From the moment they are chopped they start to lose nutrients.

- Fruits and vegetables should be eaten unpeeled wherever possible; many vitamins and minerals are concentrated just beneath the skin.

- Use frozen food if fresh is unavailable—it is nutritionally similar.

- Cut produce into large pieces rather than small; vitamins are lost from cut surfaces.

- Cook vegetables in the minimum amount of water; steaming, microwaving, or stir-frying retains the most vitamins.

- When boiling vegetables, add to fast-boiling water and cook as briefly as possible until they are tender-crisp, not soft and mushy.

- Save the water in which you've cooked veggies to make soups, stocks, and sauces.

manage to do this. Fast foods, kids' meals, processed snacks, peer pressure, and time pressure make an optimal diet very difficult to achieve. Add to this list the fact that most children miss out on the recommended five portions of fruits and vegetables daily, which means that many children may fail to reach optimal intakes of many vitamins and minerals.

A well-formulated children's multi-vitamin and -mineral supplement can help ensure that they get enough vitamins and minerals so that their growth, physical and mental development, and physical performance will remain

How to Choose a Supplement

1. Choose a comprehensive formula designed for your children's age range; ideally the following nutrients should be included: vitamin A, vitamin C, vitamin D, vitamin E, thiamin, riboflavin, niacin, vitamin B-6, folic acid, vitamin B-12, biotin, pantothenic acid, beta-carotene, calcium, phosphorus, iron, magnesium, zinc, and iodine.

2. Check that the quantities of each nutrient are no more than 100 percent of the RDA (or "Daily Value") as stated on the label.

3. Avoid supplements with added colors.

4. Try to choose brands that have been produced by established manufacturers with a good reputation for quality control and clinical research.

unimpaired. Of course, a supplement cannot take the place of a good diet, but it can give you peace of mind that your child isn't missing out on essential vitamins and minerals. Some scientists believe that the RDAs for children are inappropriate, as they have traditionally been based on preventing deficiency symptoms rather than promoting optimal health. For this reason, in the U.S. and Canada, the RDAs were updated in the last decade or so, and in most cases were increased. However, some experts still believe they're too low.

Low intakes of certain vitamins and minerals have been linked with lower IQ, poor reasoning ability, reduced physical performance, poor attention, and behavioral problems. It is possible that supplementation can help correct deficiencies and produce a significant improvement in these aspects of a child's performance. However, extra vitamins and minerals won't make children more intelligent or more athletic if they are already well nourished.

If you do decide to give your child a vitamin/mineral supplement, make sure you follow the dosage directions on the label. Additionally, don't give

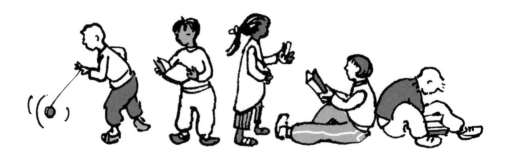

children more than one vitamin or mineral preparation (unless under medical supervision). Keep vitamin supplements well out of young children's reach; they can taste and look like candy!

Phytochemicals

Phytochemicals are plant compounds that afford particular health benefits. They include plant pigments (found in colored fruits and vegetables) and plant hormones (found in grains, beans, lentils, soy products, and herbs). Many phytochemicals work as antioxidants (see below), while others influence enzymes (such as those that block cancer agents). They offer the following benefits:

- Fight cancer
- Reduce inflammation
- Combat free radicals
- Lower cholesterol
- Reduce heart-disease risk
- Boost immunity
- Balance the intestinal flora (bacteria)
- Fight harmful bacteria and viruses

For the best protection, encourage children to eat a wide variety of different-colored foods. In general, the more intensely colored the fruit or vegetable, the greater the concentration of phytochemicals, vitamins, and minerals. You can maximize the phytochemical mix by choosing foods from each color category every day:

- Green–spinach, broccoli, cabbage, brussels sprouts, salad greens/lettuce, kale
- Red/purple–plums, eggplant, cherries, beets, red grapes, strawberries, blackberries, blueberries, tomatoes
- Yellow/orange–peaches, apricots, nectarines, oranges, yellow peppers, squash
- White/yellow–onions, garlic, apples, pears, celery
- Brown/green–beans, lentils, bean sprouts, nuts, seeds, tea

Antioxidants

Antioxidants help to protect children's bodies from the effects of free-radical damage. They include enzymes (that are made in the body), vitamins (such as beta-carotene, vitamin C, vitamin E), minerals (such as selenium), and phytochemicals. Free radicals are destructive elements that are produced all the time as a normal part of cell processes. In small numbers they are not a problem. But extra free radicals can be generated by pollution, UV sunlight, cigarette smoke, and stress. Left unchecked, they can coat and clog up the arteries and increase the risk of thrombosis, heart disease, and cancer. The good news is that antioxidants can neutralize free radicals. And an antioxidant-rich diet may help protect against these conditions and promote faster recovery after exercise.

Antioxidant nutrients are found in fruits and vegetables, seed oils, nuts, whole grains, beans, and lentils.

THE TOP ANTIOXIDANT-RICH FRUIT AND VEGETABLES[10]

Researchers at Tufts University, in Boston, have compiled the following ranking of fruits and vegetables according to their antioxidant power:

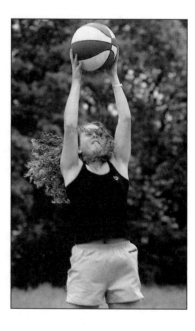

1. Prunes
2. Raisins
3. Blueberries
4. Blackberries
5. Garlic
6. Curly kale
7. Strawberries
8. Raspberries
9. Spinach
10. Brussels sprouts
11. Plums
12. Red peppers
13. Broccoli

CHAPTER 7

Eating for Action

Eating the right foods will help children to perform well in sports. A healthy diet will give them the energy they need to run, swim, cycle, and play hard, increasing their chances to reach their athletic potential. What they eat, how much they eat, and when they eat will have a big impact on their performance.

This chapter gives you practical guidelines on what children should eat before, during, and after exercise. It also deals with the practical problems of fitting meals around training times. There is often little time to eat, especially when practice sessions and exercise classes take place early in the morning or right after school. Here you'll find lots of ideas for healthy foods that can be fitted around children's busy schedules. If they are competing or traveling away from home, there's even more reason to ensure that they have the right sorts of foods and drinks available. Use the checklist and meal ideas in this chapter to make sure your kids perform at their best.

How Much Food Should My Child Eat?

Active children need more calories than their less active friends because they require extra energy to fuel their muscles for sports. This extra energy should come mainly from carbohydrate (see Chapter 4, "Carb-Charging"), with smaller amounts from protein. Therefore, plan their diet around foods high in carbohydrate, in the proportions suggested in the Food Pyramid (see Chapter 2). Keep in mind that they may need slightly larger portions of all the foods in the Food Pyramid compared with their less active friends.

Exactly how much food active children should eat is difficult to predict, but the best measure really is their appetite. Provided they are not overweight or underweight (see Chapters 9 and 10), you can safely use their appetite as a guide to portion sizes. Make sure, of course, that they are getting their extra energy from nutritious foods and not simply filling up on sugary, fatty foods.

Be guided, too, by their energy levels. If children fail to eat enough, then their energy levels will be persistently low, and they will feel lethargic and will underperform at sports. On the other hand, if they appear to have plenty of energy and get-up-and-go, then they are probably eating enough.

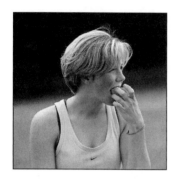

It is unrealistic to measure the calorie intake of children, but you can get a rough estimate of whether they are getting it right by checking the values in the first table below. These are the estimated requirements for average children published by the British Department of Health. These figures do not take account of regular exercise or sports, so you will need to make an allowance for your child's increased activity, if applicable.

The second table lists the estimated caloric expenditure for various activities for a ten-year-old child weighing thirty-three kilograms (about seventy-three pounds). These values are based on measurements made on adults, scaled down to the body weight of a child, with an added margin of 25 percent. (There are no published values relating to children.) The margin takes account of the relative "wastefulness" of energy in children compared with adults performing the same activity, due mainly to kids' lack of coordination. Heavier children will burn slightly more calories than the values listed in the table; lighter children will burn less.

Daily Energy Needs of Average Children		
AGE	**BOYS (CALORIES)**	**GIRLS (CALORIES)**
4–6 years	1,715	1,545
7–10 years	1,970	1,740
11–14 years	2,220	1,845

Calories Expended in Various Activities	
ACTIVITY	**CALORIES BURNED IN 30 MINUTES**
Cycling (7 mph)	88
Running (7.5 mph)	248
Sitting	24
Standing	26
Swimming (crawl, 3 mph)	353
Tennis	125
Walking	88

Values are based on measurements made on adults, scaled down to the body weight of 73 pounds (33 kg), with an added margin of 25 percent.

What Should Children Eat Before Training or Competition?

Most of the energy needed for exercise is provided by whatever children have eaten several hours or even days before. Carbohydrate in their food will have been converted into glycogen and stored in their muscles and liver (see Chapter 4). If they have eaten the right amount of carbohydrate, they will have high levels of glycogen in their muscles, ready to fuel their activity. If they have failed to eat enough carbohydrate, they will have low stocks of glycogen, putting them at risk of early fatigue during exercise.

What they eat *just before* exercise will not affect their muscle glycogen levels. Rather, it will boost their blood-glucose levels, giving them just a little more energy for their activity and possibly postponing fatigue.

Food eaten just before exercise needs to

- prevent children from feeling hungry during training
- be high in carbohydrate
- provide long-lasting energy
- be easily digested

Foods with a moderate or low GI (see Chapter 4) are best because they provide sustained energy and will help children keep going longer during

Pre-Exercise Snacks

The following foods can be eaten one to two hours before exercise along with a glass of water:

- Fresh fruit—grapes, apples, oranges, pears, bananas—and a glass of milk
- Honey spread on whole-grain bread
- Fruit bars, cereal bars, energy bars
- Yogurt and fresh fruit
- Dried fruit—raisins, apricots, mango
- Breakfast cereal with milk
- Crackers with a little cheese
- Water, diluted fruit juice (diluted 1:1), or sports drink
- Crackers and rice cakes with bananas or honey
- Rolls, sandwiches, English muffins, mini bagels, mini pancakes
- Homemade muffins and cakes (see recipes on pages 194–199)

exercise. Don't let them eat lots of sugary foods such as sweets and soft drinks just before exercising. Doing so may cause a quick surge of blood glucose, followed by a sharp fall, which will leave them lacking in energy and unable to keep going at a good pace.

Avoid high-fat foods as well, because they empty from the stomach too slowly. A high-fat snack could make children feel uncomfortable and sick during practice or an event. Fats eaten before exercise do not raise blood glucose levels, so they will not benefit performance. So what is best? Either a low-GI carbohydrate food (e.g., fresh fruit or pasta), or a protein combined with a high-GI carbohydrate food (e.g., breakfast cereal with milk) will produce sustained energy. The boxes below give some ideas for suitable pre-exercise snacks and meals. It takes a certain amount of trial and error to find out which foods suit an individual child best and exactly how much to eat. Use the box as a guide to the right kinds of foods. Adjust the quantities according to kids' appetite, how they feel, and what they like. It's important that they feel comfortable with the types and amounts of foods they're eating. Don't offer anything new before a competition, as it may not agree with them. Drinking is, of course, very important before exercise, so make sure children have a glass of water or diluted fruit juice fifteen to thirty minutes before training or competing. See Chapter 8 for more details on drinking.

Pre-Exercise Meals

The following foods can be eaten two to three hours before exercise along with a glass of water:

- Sandwich/roll filled with tuna, cheese, chicken, or peanut butter
- Baked potato with cheese, tuna, or baked beans
- Pasta with tomato-based sauce and fish or beans
- Rice or noodles with chicken or dried beans/legumes
- Breakfast cereal with milk and banana
- Hot cereal with raisins
- Lentil/vegetable or chicken soup with whole-grain bread
- Veggie or chicken burrito with beans, cheese, lettuce, tomato, on corn or flour tortilla

Timing the Pre-Exercise Meal

The timing of the pre-exercise meal may depend on practical constraints; for example, your child's class or practice may be right after school, leaving little time to eat. If there is less than one hour between eating and training, give them a light snack (see "Pre-Exercise Snacks" on the previous page). If they have more than two hours between eating and training, a normal balanced meal is suitable. This should be based around a carbohydrate food such as bread or potatoes together with a little protein such as chicken or beans, as well as a portion of vegetables and a drink (see "Pre-Exercise Meals" above).

Eating Before an Event

If they are competing, you need to make sure that children have access to the right kinds of food. It's usually a good idea to take a supply of food with you, as suitable foods and drinks may not be available at the event venue.

Children should have their normal meal about two to three hours before the event, allowing enough time to digest the food and for the stomach to empty. For example, if the event is in the morning, schedule breakfast two to three hours before the event's starting time. Similarly, if the event is in the afternoon, adjust the timing of lunch to two or three hours before the event.

Children may feel too nervous or excited to eat on the day of the event. In that case, offer nutritious drinks (such as diluted fruit juice or sports drinks), milkshakes, or light snacks. If they skip meals children may become light-headed or nauseous during the event and will not perform at their best. Here are some simple rules to follow on the day of the event:

- Do not eat or drink anything new
- Stick to familiar foods and drinks
- Take your own foods and drinks whenever possible
- Drink plenty of water or diluted juice before and after the event (see Chapter 8, "Drinking for Action")
- Eat high-carbohydrate snacks (see box "Pre-Exercise Snacks")
- Avoid high-fat foods before the event
- Avoid eating sweets and chocolates during the hour before the event
- Avoid soft drinks (containing more than 6 g sugar/100 ml) an hour before the event
- Encourage children to go to the toilet just before the event

What Should Children Eat During Exercise?

If children will be exercising continually for less than ninety minutes, they won't need to eat anything during exercise. They should, however, be encouraged to take regular drink breaks, ideally every fifteen to twenty minutes or whenever there is a suitable break in training or play. Make sure they take a water bottle and keep it within easy reach, for example, at the poolside, at the side of the soccer field, or by the track (see Chapter 8, "Drinking for Action," page 70).

During an all-day training session or competition, have food and drink available during the short breaks. For example, make opportunities to refuel

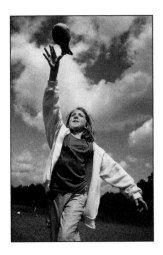

between swimming heats, tennis games, and gymnastic events. During matches or tournaments lasting more than an hour (e.g., soccer, baseball, or hockey), offer them food and drink during the half-time interval or between innings.

What types of foods should kids eat during exercise? High-carbohydrate foods and beverages are the obvious choice, as these will help to keep up their energy, maintain their blood-glucose levels, delay the onset of fatigue, and prevent hypoglycemia (low blood-glucose levels). Foods and drinks similar to those eaten before training or competition are suitable. The important thing is that they are easily digested, high in carbohydrate, and low in fat. As you will almost certainly need to take them with you, they should also be nonperishable, portable, and quick and easy to eat. Sometimes food is provided at events, but you will need to find out beforehand exactly what will be available—it may be simply chips, chocolate bars, and soft drinks, all of which are unhelpful for good performance! Check the box below for suitable snacks.

Snacks for Short Breaks During Training or Competition

- Water, diluted fruit juice, sports drinks

- Bananas

- Fresh fruit—grapes, apples, oranges, pears

- Dried fruit—raisins, apricots, mangoes

- Crackers and rice cakes with bananas or honey

- Rolls, sandwiches, English muffins, mini bagels, mini pancakes

- Fruit bars, cereal bars, energy bars

What Should Children Eat after Exercise?

After exercise, the first priority is to replenish fluid losses. So give children a drink right away—water or diluted fruit juice are the best choices (see Chapter 8, "Drinking for Action").

Suitable Recovery Snacks

Accompany all snacks with a drink of water or diluted fruit juice.

- Fresh fruit, e.g., bananas, grapes, apples
- Dried fruit
- Fruit yogurt
- Yogurt drink
- Smoothie (see recipes on pages 202–206)
- Roll or bagel with jam or honey
- Mini pancakes
- Homemade muffins, snack bars, cookies (see recipes on pages 194–201)
- Homemade apple, carrot, or fruit cake (see recipes on pages 196–199)
- Homemade milkshake (see recipes on pages 202–206)

Children also need to replace the energy they have just used. It's rather like refilling your gas tank after completing a long journey. And the sooner they eat carbohydrate, the faster they will replenish their energy stores. That's because the body is most efficient at converting carbohydrate into glycogen in the muscles during the first two hours after exercise. In fact, the postexercise snack or meal is perhaps the most important meal as it determines how fast children will recover before the next training session. Unless they will be eating a meal within half an hour, give them a snack to stave off hunger and promote recovery. The exact amounts you should provide will depend on children's appetite and body size. As a guide, give just enough to alleviate their hunger and keep them going until mealtime. Studies with adult athletes have shown that one gram of carbohydrate per kilogram of body weight eaten within two hours of exercise speeds recovery. (To determine body weight in kilograms, divide weight in pounds by 2.2.)

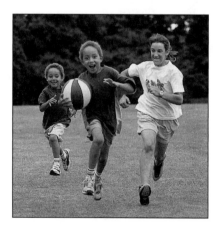

So, what are the best foods to eat after exercise? High-carbohydrate foods with a moder-

Suitable Recovery Meals

Accompany all meals with a drink of water or diluted fruit juice and one or two portions of vegetables or salad.

- Baked potatoes with beans, tuna, or cheese

- Pasta with tomato sauce and cheese

- Rice with chicken and stir-fried vegetables

- Hummus on a bagel

- Veggie or chicken burrito with beans, cheese, lettuce, tomato, on a corn or flour tortilla

ate or high GI should be included in this recovery snack or meal. They will raise blood-glucose levels fairly rapidly and then be converted quickly into glycogen in the muscles. Recent studies with adult athletes have found that including a little protein (in a ratio of about 3:1 carbohydrate to protein) enhances recovery further. Check the box below for suitable recovery snacks and meals. Unfortunately, most of the snacks on offer in the snack bar or vending machines at sports clubs and venues are highly unsuitable; however, this is changing in some places. Foods such as chips, chocolate bars, candy, and soft drinks do not promote good recovery after exercise. They are little more than concentrated forms of sugar, fat, or salt, and actually slow down rehydration. Because they also provide a lot of calories, these foods can take away your child's appetite for healthier foods at the next meal. So what can you do? Let the venue know that you are unhappy with the choice of snacks on offer to children, ask other parents and coaches to do the same, and suggest that they replace these "junk" foods with healthier choices. Even better, show this chapter to the folks who run the snack bar. Any of the suggestions in the box titled "Suitable Recovery Snacks" would be appropriate offerings for kids after a sporting event. As an interim measure, encourage children to take their own drinks and snacks.

Traveling and Competing Away from Home

When children are traveling to compete away from home, organize their food and beverages in advance and take them with you. They may need

Snacks for Eating on the Move

- Sandwiches filled with chicken or tuna or cheese with lettuce and tomato; banana and peanut butter sandwiches
- Rice cakes, oat cakes, whole-grain crackers
- Bottles of water
- Cartons of fruit juice
- Yogurt drinks
- Individual cheese portions
- Small bags of nuts—peanuts, cashews, almonds
- Fresh fruit—apples, bananas, grapes
- Mini boxes of raisins
- Fruit bar or energy bar
- Prepared vegetable crudités (e.g., carrots, peppers, cucumber, celery)

snacks for the journey, so take a supply of suitable foods; use any of the suggestions in the box titled "Snacks for Eating on the Move." Do not rely on roadside cafes, fast-food restaurants, or airport catering outlets; healthy choices are often limited at these places. Make sure you take plenty of drinks, in case of delays. Air-conditioned travel in cars and planes can quickly make children dehydrated.

Try to find out what catering arrangements have been made at the venue. Check the local restaurants and takeaway stands. Encourage children to choose dishes that are high in carbohydrate, such as pasta, pizza, or rice dishes. And warn them against trying anything unfamiliar or unusual–the last thing they need is an upset stomach before the event! When traveling abroad it's best to avoid common food-poisoning culprits–such as chicken, seafood, and meat dishes–unless you are sure they have been properly cooked and heated to a high temperature. Be wary of such foods served lukewarm. Check the box titled "Suitable Restaurant Meals and Fast Foods when Traveling to a Sports Event," below, for ideas about meals away from home.

Remember, too, that children will probably feel nervous or apprehensive when traveling. They may not feel like eating much food. In this case, encourage them to drink plenty of nutritious beverages instead, such as fruit juice, smoothies, yogurt drinks, and milkshakes. Pack their favorite foods–of the nonperishable variety–to tempt their appetite. Sometimes it's a case of simply getting them to eat something rather than nothing. If they stop eating they will run down their energy reserves, putting them at a disadvantage for competition.

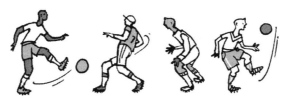

Suitable Restaurant Meals and Fast Foods when Traveling to a Sports Event

- Simple pasta dishes with tomato sauce
- Rice and stir-fried vegetable dishes
- Pizza with tomato and vegetable toppings
- Simple noodle dishes
- Baked potatoes with cheese
- Pancakes with syrup or fruit or yogurt
- Veggie or chicken burrito

Restaurant Meals and Fast Foods to Avoid

- Burgers and fries
- Chicken nuggets
- Pasta with creamy or oily sauces
- Fatty Mexican foods
- Fried fish and chips
- Lukewarm chicken, turkey, meat, fish, or seafood dishes
- Hot dogs
- Fried chicken meals

CHAPTER 8

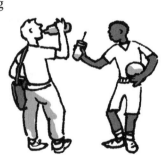

Drinking for Action

Drinking is just as important as eating. Not only is water essential for keeping children alive and functioning normally, but it also makes a big difference in their physical performance. If children become even mildly dehydrated during exercise they will start to feel unwell and be unable to perform at their best. In fact, early signs of dehydration are easily missed in children, so this chapter tells you what to look out for and how to prevent your child from becoming dehydrated during exercise. It also explains which beverages are best for children who exercise and whether soft drinks and sports drinks are worthwhile. After all, today there is a bewildering choice of beverages targeted at children. It's also important to know how much they should drink before and during exercise; this chapter offers some simple guidelines on the amount and timing of drinking around exercise.

Why Is Drinking Important for My Child?

Children are much more susceptible to dehydration and overheating than adults for the following reasons:

- They sweat less than adults (sweat helps to keep the body's temperature stable).

- They cannot cope with very hot conditions as well as adults.

- They get hotter during exercise.
- Their bodies have a greater surface area for their weight.
- They often fail to recognize or respond to feelings of thirst.

By the time children are thirsty they have already lost quite a bit of fluid and may already be dehydrated. Dehydration can set in when they have lost as little as 1 percent of their body weight. For a ten-year-old weighing 75 pounds, that would be a mere three-quarters of a pound.

Apart from increased body temperature, there are other side effects of dehydration:

- Exercise feels much harder
- Heart rate increases more than usual
- May develop cramps, headache, and nausea
- Concentration is reduced
- Ability to perform sports skills drops
- Fatigues sooner and loses stamina

Six Ways to Keep Cool

1. Provide extra water during hot and humid weather.
2. Schedule exercise for the cooler times of the day during hot weather.
3. Schedule regular drink breaks during activity, ideally in the shade during hot weather.
4. Encourage children to wear loose-fitting, natural-fiber clothing during exercise that allows them to sweat freely and permits moisture to evaporate.
5. Let them acclimatize gradually to hot or humid weather conditions; allow two weeks.
6. Make sure kids drink extra water during the twenty-four hours before a competition.

It is impossible for children (and adults!) to perform at their best when they are dehydrated. You cannot and should not train children to tolerate exercising without drinking. A few sports coaches still restrict fluids during training, in the misguided belief that the human body will eventually adapt to low fluid intakes, or perhaps simply to remove the hassle and distraction of drinking itself! However, even if children manage to exercise under such conditions, they will be performing below par. They will also be at risk of developing heat cramps and heat exhaustion.

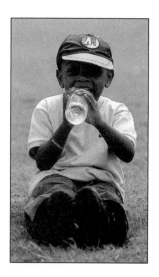

Dehydration Check-Up

One of the most reliable tests for dehydration is the "pee test"—checking the color, volume, and odor of the urine. If it is almost clear or very pale yellow and the child needs to pass urine quite frequently (about once every one or two hours), the level of hydration is good. The more intensely colored it is, the greater the degree of dehydration. Smaller than usual volumes of very yellow or gold-colored urine, for example, would indicate that the child is dehydrated and should drink extra water until the urine becomes paler.

How Much Should Children Drink?

Children need to drink enough fluid to prevent dehydration. On average, children will lose between 350 and 700 milliliters of body fluid (1½ to 2½ cups; equivalent to 0.75 to 1.5 pounds of body weight) during an hour's exercise. If it's hot and humid or they are wearing lots of layers of clothing, they will sweat more and lose even more fluid.

To replace the lost fluid, children must drink plenty of fluid before, during, and after exercise. The exact amount depends on the following:

- The temperature and humidity of the surroundings—the warmer and higher the humidity, the greater their sweat losses and the more they will need to drink.

- How hard they are exercising—the harder they exercise, the more they will sweat and the more they will need to drink.

- How long they are exercising—the longer they exercise, the more they will sweat and the more they will need to drink.

Warning Signs of Dehydration

Children can become dehydrated more easily than adults. Here are some of the signs to look out for.

Early symptoms

- Unusually lacking in energy
- Fatiguing early during exercise
- Complaining of feeling too hot
- Skin appears flushed and feels clammy
- Passing only small volumes of dark-colored urine
- Nausea

Action: Drink 100–200 ml (½ to ¾ cup) water or sports drink every ten to fifteen minutes.

Advanced symptoms

- A bad headache
- Becomes dizzy or light-headed
- Appears disorientated
- Short of breath (more so than usual)

Action: Drink 100–200 ml (½ to ¾ cup) sports drink every ten to fifteen minutes (in case of advanced symptoms, sports drinks are a must; water is not sufficient). Seek professional help.

- Their size—the bigger they are, the more they will sweat and the more they will need to drink.
- Their fitness—the fitter they are, the earlier and more profusely they sweat (it's a sign of good body-temperature control) and the more they will need to drink (especially compared to their less-fit friends).

Make sure that children are well hydrated before exercise (see "Dehydration Check-Up," above). If they are slightly dehydrated at this stage there is a bigger risk of overheating once they start exercising. Encourage them to drink six to eight cups (1 to 1¹/₂ liters) of fluid during the day and, as a final measure, to top up with ³/₄–1 cup of water forty-five minutes before exercise.

You can estimate how much fluid children have lost during exercise by weighing them before and after a session. For each 1 kilogram (2.2 pounds) lost, they should drink 1¹/₂ liters (approximately 1¹/₂ quarts) of fluid. This accounts for the fact that they continue to sweat after exercise and also to lose more fluid through urine. For example, if a child weighs 0.3 kg (²/₃ pound) less after exercise, he has lost 0.3 liters (300 ml; about 1¹/₃ cup) of fluid. To replace 300 ml of fluid he needs to drink 300 X 1¹/₂ = 450 ml of fluid (about 2 cups). But don't expect children to drink large volumes after exercising. Divide their drinks into manageable amounts to be taken during and after exercise. A good strategy would be to drink, say, 100 ml (¹/₂ cup) at three regular intervals during exercise, then 150 ml afterwards.

Use the following guidelines, in conjunction with the above considerations, to plan your children's drinking strategy:

BEFORE EXERCISE	DURING EXERCISE	AFTER EXERCISE
150–200 ml (³/₄–1 cup) 45 minutes before activity	75–100 ml (about ¹/₂ cup) every 15–20 minutes	Drink freely until no longer thirsty, plus an extra glass; or drink 300 ml (about 1 ¹/₃ cup) for every 0.2 kg (¹/₂ pound) weight loss

How to Fit It All In

Fitting in six to eight glasses of water a day isn't difficult once children get into the habit of drinking regularly. They could have a glass of water or diluted fruit juice first thing in the morning. Also encourage them to drink a glass of water, diluted juice, or milk with each meal (see the list of recommended drinks on page 202), a glass between meals, and perhaps a final glass of water last thing at night. It may be more convenient to carry a drinking bottle so that a few sips are never far away.

How to Make Children Drink while Exercising

- Make drinking more fun with a novelty water bottle.

- Make sure they place the bottle within easy access, e.g., at one end of the pool or by the side of the track, court, gym, or field.

- Encourage them to take regular sips, ideally every ten to twenty minutes. This may take practice.

- Tell them not to wait until they are thirsty. Plan a drink during the first twenty minutes of exercise, then at regular intervals during the session, even if they don't "feel" thirsty.

- If they are playing a team sport, have them think ahead about suitable drink breaks, e.g., at halftime during a game, or while listening to the coach during practice sessions.

- If they don't like water, offer a flavored drink such as diluted fruit juice or a sports drink (see "What Should Children Drink?" below).

- Slightly chilling the beverage (to around 40°F) usually encourages children to drink more.

What Should Children Drink?

Plain water is best for most activities lasting less than ninety minutes. It replaces lost fluids rapidly and so makes a perfectly good drink for sports.

But there are two potential problems with drinking water. First, many children are unexcited about drinking water, so they simply fail to drink enough. Second, water tends to quench one's thirst even though the body is still dehydrated.

Encourage water whenever possible, but if your children find it difficult to drink enough water, give them a flavored drink. Diluted fruit juice (two parts water to one part juice) or isotonic sports drinks are options. Although these beverages probably won't benefit children's performance for activities lasting less than ninety minutes, they will encourage kids to drink larger volumes of fluid. But observe a word of caution about commercial sports drinks: in practice, many children find that sports drinks sit "heavily" in their stomachs. If that is the case, you may either dilute the sports drink with

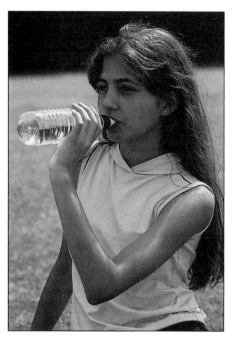

water (if making it from powder, add a little extra water), or alternate sports drinks with water.

If children will be exercising hard and continuously for more than ninety minutes, sports drinks containing around 4–6 g of sugars per 100 ml may benefit their performance. This is because the sugars in these drinks help fuel the exercising muscles and postpone fatigue. The electrolytes (sodium and potassium) contained in the drinks are designed to stimulate thirst and make them drink more. Also, at the right dilution (4–6 g/100 ml), these sugars help the body absorb water faster. And the faster you can get water back into the body, the better. Always check the sugar content, though. If the drink is too concentrated (more than 6–8 g sugars/100 ml) the drink will stay in the stomach longer (making your child feel uncomfortable), and it will take longer to get absorbed (possibly exacerbating dehydration).

On the downside, sports drinks are relatively expensive. It's cheaper to make your own version by diluting fruit juice (one part juice to one or two

What Children Shouldn't Drink!

- Fizzy drinks—the bubbles in fizzy drinks may cause a burning sensation in the mouth, especially if drunk quickly, and will certainly stop children from drinking enough fluid. Fizzy drinks can also upset the stomach and make kids' feel bloated and uncomfortable during exercise.

- Soft drinks—these are too concentrated in sugar and will tend to sit in the stomach too long during exercise. They may make children feel nauseous and uncomfortable.

- Drinks containing caffeine—including caffeinated soft drinks, coffee, and tea. Caffeine dehydrates the body even more. It may also increase the heart rate and cause trembling, as children are more sensitive to caffeine than adults.

parts water) or organic fruit punch (diluted one part punch to six parts water). The fruit-juice version would also help maintain energy levels (blood glucose) during prolonged exercise.

The most important thing is that children drink enough. Therefore, the taste is important. If they don't like it, they won't drink it! Experiment with different flavors until you find the ones they like. A little trial and error may also be needed to find the best concentration. If it's too concentrated, it will sit in kids' stomachs and make them feel uncomfortable.

Choosing the Best Drink for Exercise

EXERCISE LASTING LESS THAN 90 MINUTES	EXERCISE LASTING MORE THAN 90 MINUTES
Water	Sports drink (4–6 g sugars/100 ml)
Fruit juice diluted 2 parts water to 1 part juice	Fruit juice diluted 1–2 parts water to 1 part juice
Sports drink alternated with water	Fruit punch (ideally organic) diluted 6 parts water to 1 part punch

CHAPTER 9

🌶🥕🫑🍊🍄🍓

Overweight Kids

There is little doubt that overweight children are more common nowadays than in generations past. Fifteen percent of American children and teens ages six to nineteen (roughly nine million) are overweight, according to data

from a national study conducted in 1999–2000. This is triple what the proportion was in 1980. The same survey showed that another 15 percent of kids in this age range are considered at risk for becoming overweight. In addition, over 10 percent of children between the ages of two and five are overweight, up from 7 percent in 1994.[11]

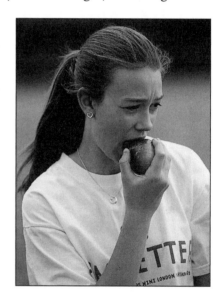

This chapter looks at the reasons why so many children are overweight and offers practical advice on what you can do about it. Clearly, being overweight affects children's health now and in the future. It also affects their physical performance and self-esteem. Overweight children are more likely to become overweight adults.

Dieting is not the answer. No one wants to see children on fad diets, ruining their health. But at the same time, you cannot sit back and do nothing. This chapter details key strategies to help you deal with children's weight problems.

What Are the Dangers for Children of Being Overweight?

Although the immediate medical risks of being overweight as a child are small, research has highlighted the following risks for overweight children:

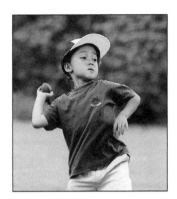

- Bone and joint problems—knee, hip, and foot problems may develop due to the burden of supporting extra weight
- Breathing problems, particularly at night and during exertion
- High blood pressure
- High blood cholesterol
- Artery damage and increased risk of heart disease in adulthood

Perhaps the biggest health hazard is that overweight kids are more likely to grow into overweight adults. And with being overweight in adulthood comes obesity-related diseases, such as type-II diabetes, heart disease, and stroke. Most overweight adults were overweight as children. An Australian study of obese eighteen-year-olds found that 90 percent were obese at the age of nine. It also found that being overweight tends to go hand in hand with inactivity and a low level of fitness.[12] What's certain is that poor eating and exercise habits established during childhood are likely to persist. It's more difficult to lose weight or to take up sports as an adult than as a child. That means now is the time to act. If children can be encouraged to eat more healthily and to get more exercise, they will avoid obesity and more serious problems in adulthood.

Fat Parents = Fat Kids?

Children with overweight parents are more likely to be fat themselves. A study at the Institute of Child Health in London found that seven-year-old girls with two overweight parents were 10 percent heavier than those with parents in the normal weight range. By the age of thirteen, the difference had risen to 20 percent. A study at Liverpool's Institute of Child Health revealed that children who are more than slightly overweight by the age of seven have a 60 percent chance of being obese when they are fourteen to sixteen years old.[13]

Heart Symptoms in Obese Children

One of the most worrisome findings among obese children is the sign of artery damage. In 2001, researchers at the Armand-Trousseau Hospital in Paris found that the arteries of obese children were much stiffer and more damaged than those of normal-weight children. This puts them at greater risk of heart disease and stroke in later life.

How Can I Tell If a Child Is Overweight?

The easiest way to tell whether children are overweight is by comparing them with their friends of a similar age. Seeing kids next to each other in their sports uniforms or swimsuits can reveal big differences in body size and body fat.

But often children know they are fat; they are told so by other children. Cruel though this is, if they are teased about their weight at school, it is probably confirmation that they have a weight problem. They may find it hard to take part in sports or other school activities, or may be unable to wear the same clothes as other children. They will begin to feel differently about themselves and may start to feel unhappy.

Sometimes whether a child is overweight is not clear-cut. In some cases it can be difficult to know whether children are just gearing up for a growth spurt, or whether you are projecting your own worries about weight onto a perfectly normal child. A stocky or "big-boned" child is probably fine. But if their tummy hangs over the waistband of their trousers, then you may have reason for concern. Height and weight charts only tell you about average children. They don't account for children with different body types, nor do they tell you how much fat an individual child has.

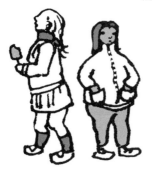

You can perform the pinch test to get a rough idea of how much excess fat a child has. It's not as accurate as skin-fold calipers (used for measuring the amount of body fat in adults) but will alert you as to whether you need to take action. Using your thumb and forefinger, see how much excess fat you can pinch just above the hipbones, around the belly button, or on the lower back. If it's more than an inch, then now is the time to talk to your child about activity and healthy eating.

Overweight or Obese?

Being overweight is defined as having a body mass index (BMI) greater than the norm for that age. A normal BMI is between 17.2 and 23.9, depending on age and gender. Obesity is defined as being significantly over the normal BMI (above 19.2–29.1, depending on age and gender).

Use the following steps to calculate the BMI:

1. Divide your weight in pounds by your height in inches.

2. Divide that number again by your height in inches.

3. Multiply that number by 703.

For example, a child weighing 140 pounds and measuring 65 inches would have a BMI of 23.27, calculated as follows:

Step 1: 140 (weight) ÷ 65 (height) = 2.154

Step 2: 2.154 ÷ 65 (height)= 0.0331

Step 3: 0.0331 x 703 = 23.27 (BMI)

BMIs for Overweight or Obese Children				
AGE	**OVERWEIGHT**		**OBESE**	
	Boys	Girls	Boys	Girls
5	≥17.4	≥17.2	≥19.3	≥19.2
7	≥17.9	≥17.8	≥20.6	≥20.5
10	≥19.8	≥19.9	≥24.0	≥24.1
12	≥21.2	≥21.7	≥26.0	≥26.7
15	≥23.3	≥23.9	≥28.3	≥29.1

Why Do Children Become Overweight?

Simply put, children become overweight when there is a mismatch between calorie intake and calorie output. In other words, more calories are consumed from food than are burned during activity. There may be several reasons why this mismatch happens. The key ones are the following:

- Heredity
- Overeating
- Lack of physical activity

Let's look at each factor a little more closely.

HEREDITY

If you look objectively at children's basic body shapes and then compare them with their parent's body shapes, you will probably notice a striking similarity. Children's body shapes tend to bear a close resemblance to that of one of their parents. Just as they inherit blue eyes or brown hair, they can inherit a body type that has a greater tendency to put on weight. This is called the *endomorphic* body type (see the box titled "Body Types").

Does this mean that you can inherit being overweight? Well, studies have shown that children of two obese parents have an 80 percent chance of being obese, a 40 percent chance if only one parent is obese, and yet only a 3 percent chance if both parents are lean. Studies with identical twins who were adopted by different parents have found that the weights and shapes of the identical twins remained remarkably similar even though they were brought up in different homes.[14]

So it seems as if you can inherit a greater tendency to gain weight. Indeed, scientists have identified several genes that govern appetite and metabolic rate. But—and this is a big but—even if children have inherited a tendency to gain fat, being overweight is by no means inevitable. With a positive attitude, good nutrition habits, and regular activity, they can maintain a sensible weight.

Body Types

Anthropologists use three main body-type classifications: the ectomorph, the mesomorph, and the endomorph. The ectomorph tends to be tall, long-limbed, and thin. The mesomorph tends to be naturally muscular with an athletic frame. The endomorph has a more rounded frame with a greater tendency to put on excess weight. Few people fit one body type perfectly, but everyone has a tendency toward one (or two) body types. Therefore, if a child has mostly endomorphic characteristics, the chances are they have inherited those characteristics from one or both parents.

OVEREATING

Many overweight children appear to eat less food than their friends, yet they remain overweight. In fact, it's not the amount–or volume–of food that matters; it's what they eat and how often they eat.

Look carefully at the kinds of food kids eat and how frequently they eat them. Count the number of times they indulge in snack foods such as chips, chocolate, cookies, candy, and pastries each day. Do they get regular lunchbox treats? What do they eat after school? Do they regularly eat sugary or high-fat snacks in front of the television? Do they rely on fast foods and "kiddie" meals such as fries, burgers, nuggets, and tacos? How often do they drink sugar-laden soft drinks and fruit punches? The problem with all of these kinds of foods is that they are dense in calories–that is, they are full of fat and/or sugar, they contain very little fiber and little water, and they have very little "filling power" and so are easy to overeat. Just think how easy it is to quickly scarf down a few cookies in front of the TV. They quickly add up to a few hundred calories, which, unless used to fuel physical activity, will be stored as fat. Soft drinks are a big culprit. They are high in sugar yet not very filling, and so can add a lot of unwanted calories to children's diets. A diet comprising these kinds of foods and beverages is a recipe for disaster.

The solution is not necessarily to ban these foods completely. Rather, limit sugary and fatty foods and encourage children to try more nutritious and filling foods. You can instill good eating habits without banning "treat" foods altogether (see "What Practical Help Can I Give?"on page 85).

LACK OF PHYSICAL ACTIVITY

Lack of exercise and activity are big problems with many children, whether overweight or not. Combined with unhealthy eating habits, inactivity will certainly lead to overweight. How much time do your children spend sitting–at school, at home, in front of the television, or at the computer? If they are sitting in front of the TV or computer, it means they are not running around and getting exercise. Worse still, television watching lowers the metabolism (the number of calories burned) to barely baseline levels. Researchers have shown that children watching television burn fewer calories than if they were reading or drawing a picture! Television induces an almost trancelike state in children, reducing their energy output to a bare minimum.

How much physical activity do your children engage in at school? It may be less than you think. There are fewer compulsory sports and PE classes than ever before. Faced with restricted budgets, more and more schools are eliminating or reducing recess and PE, the result being that many children get very little exercise during school hours.

Are your children driven to school? A generation ago, most children walked or cycled to school, but now traffic congestion and fears for child safety mean that many children are missing out on another opportunity for physical activity. It's common to see children being driven everywhere else, too. Pressures of time mean that many children don't make a habit of walking or cycling.

Glued to the Television?

Many experts blame weight problems on too much television. It replaces exercise, significantly lowers the metabolism, encourages unhealthy snacking, and increases children's exposure to junk-food ads. A four-year study at the Harvard School of Public Health compared the heights and weights of 786 children aged between six and eleven. Those who watched more than five hours of TV a day were more than four times as likely to be overweight as those who watched two hours or less a day.

How Should I Deal with Children's Weight Problems?

Don't tell children that they should lose weight, even if you are concerned about their weight. Don't punish or scold children—use positive reinforcement. It is important to emphasize feeling healthy and strong. No matter what their size and shape, help them love themselves by praising their strengths and skills. As a parent, reassure them that your love for them is not conditional on how they look or how much they weigh. However, it is important to recognize a weight problem early. Don't sit back and hope that children will "grow out of it." The longer a child is overweight, the more difficult it will be to establish a healthy weight. So what's the first step?

For children who are only moderately overweight, don't expect them to lose weight, as this could compromise their growth and development. Rather, the goal should be weight maintenance rather than weight loss, allowing children to "grow into" their weight as they get taller. The more slowly this happens, the more likely they will be able to maintain it. Never put children on a "slimming diet"; they could miss out on essential nutrients and fail to grow normally. Nor should you feed them different meals from what the rest of the family eats; doing so will cause them to feel more self-conscious about their weight and more likely to rebel against eating healthily. You can help stall their weight gain by concentrating on an overall change toward a healthy lifestyle. Try to approach it in a low-key way, talking about healthy eating rather than "'dieting," and never labeling them as "fat." The situation is even more delicate with girls, as they are more likely than boys to become obsessed with their weight. Girls, in particular, are bombarded by the media and advertisements with images promoting slim as beautiful. So it's important that you play down your concerns about your child's or even your own weight.

For children who are very overweight, ask your doctor for advice and a referral to a registered dietitian (RD). A medically supervised weight-loss program may be suggested, but the emphasis should be on adopting a healthier lifestyle for the long term.

What Practical Help Can I Give?

To promote a healthy lifestyle, children should be encouraged to

- increase their physical activity
- adopt healthier eating habits
- reduce the time spent doing sedentary activities

Think of it as a long-term change rather than a quick fix. Here are some general guidelines:

- Be a role model—they should see that you exercise and eat a balanced diet.
- Encourage the whole family to make healthy food choices and become more active rather than singling out your overweight child.
- Do not impose restrictions on their eating habits that are different from those of other family members.

- Limit TV viewing and computer time for the whole family. Don't eat in front of the TV.
- Always talk about food in a positive way and discourage talk about weight unless the child brings it up.

How Can Children Be Encouraged to Be More Active?

Make plenty of opportunities for children to be active, and give them plenty of support and encouragement. Let them know that exercise is important in everyone's life and should be part of the daily routine. Think of this as a change for the whole family and don't put the focus on your overweight child. Seize daily opportunities to get your family moving, and build these into the daily routine. For example:

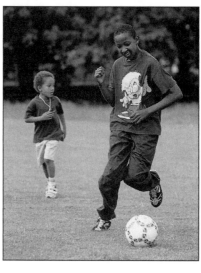

- Walk to and from school and other local places, whenever possible.
- Use the stairs rather than the elevator.
- Schedule a family swim or bike ride on weekends.
- When you do drive somewhere, park a few blocks away from your destination and walk the last part.

Try to limit the amount of time spent doing passive and sedentary activities, such as watching television and playing computer games. Sedentary activity needs to be balanced with physical activity.

Help children to do more strenuous physical activity. It doesn't matter what it is, provided it lasts for at least twenty minutes and they enjoy it: dancing, cycling, swimming, skating, and playing outdoor games such as tag are all great forms of exercise and good fun. Respect your children's individuality and let them make their own choices about exercise as much as possible. For example, let them choose which sport or activity they would like to try; do not force them to take lessons in a particular sport if they dislike it.

Here are some tips for getting kids moving:

- Set an example—they will notice whether you lead a physically active lifestyle. Children are more likely to copy what you do than what you say.

- Look for ways to incorporate activity into everything you do, and make this as much fun as possible. Turn activity into games or social activities.

- Walk or cycle with them to and from school—that will benefit both your children and you, and will show them that you are active too.

- For kids under eleven, provide plenty of play equipment at home—balls, trampolines, basketball hoops, scooters, bikes, skates, and jump ropes.

- Encourage them to enjoy a wide range of sports—soccer, baseball or softball, informal racket games, gymnastics, dance lessons, trampolining, and swimming are all suitable for children under eleven. For older children, organized sports, roller-skating, hockey, tennis, badminton, volleyball, jogging, and sailing are also suitable.

- They should pick activities they enjoy; having fun is the key to exercising for life.

How Much Exercise Should Children Get?

Children aged six to ten years should do sixty minutes of moderate-intensity activity as part of their lifestyle every day. Children aged eleven to fifteen years should do thirty to sixty minutes of moderate to vigorous activity every day as part of their lifestyle. For both age groups, this recommendation can include everyday activities such as walking, unstructured play such as ball games, chase, and hide and seek, as well as formal sports activities and PE class. For kids under eleven, their total activity time can be broken down into several sessions—for example two fifteen-minute activities in the morning, plus half an hour of activity in the afternoon; it doesn't have to be done in one session. Children aged eleven to fifteen years should aim for three sessions per week of continuous vigorous activity lasting at least twenty minutes. These could include jogging, swimming, cycling, dancing, soccer, or basketball.

How Much Exercise Do Children Really Get?

Children may appear to be playing lots of sports but may not, in fact, be getting much exercise. Observe what they are actually doing during practice. For example, during baseball and softball they often spend a lot of time standing or doing very low intensity activity—not enough to build their fitness or manage their weight. If they play team sports such as soccer, hockey, or volleyball, find out whether they spend most of the time sitting on the bench in reserve or playing goalie. If either is the case, ask the teacher or coach if they can be moved to other positions, or help children select alternative activities that they are better suited to and that they enjoy.

How Can Children Adopt Healthier Eating Habits?

The best that you can do is to offer them information and help. Talk to them about healthy eating, discuss the foods you buy and plan to eat, and then trust children to make the right choices.

Create healthy habits for the whole family, and make mealtimes enjoyable and stress-free. Make sure you do not discuss family conflicts, weight issues, or eating habits at the meal table. No foods should be forbidden or labeled in a negative way, as this could make children crave "bad" foods even more and then 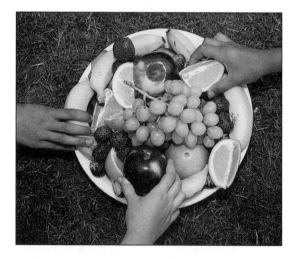 make them feel guilty when they eat them. Explain that all foods are allowed in a healthy diet, but certain ones should be eaten only occasionally or kept as occasional treats. Never give food as a reward or withhold it as a punishment. Encourage children to eat slowly and to enjoy all foods–even those occasional treats. Discourage secretive eating, overeating, or eating too fast.

Here are some specific strategies:

- Offer only healthy snacks (see box below), and keep them in a place where children can easily get them.
- Eliminate unhealthy foods from your household–remove the temptation for everyone in the family.
- Limit foods high in saturated fats and hydrogenated fats: butter, fried foods, fast foods, cookies, pastries, chocolate, cakes, chips, and other snacks.
- Use lower-fat cooking methods for family meals.
- Eat foods in the proportions suggested in the Food Pyramid (see Chapter 2), adjusting the portion sizes if necessary.
- Emphasize grains (six to eight portions), fresh fruit (two to four portions), and vegetables (three to five portions) in family meals (see the recipes in Chapter 14).
- Offer three nutritious meals a day.

Nutritious Snacks

- Whole-grain crackers
- Whole-grain toast with peanut butter or honey
- Fresh fruit (e.g., apple slices, oranges, tangerines, grapes, strawberries, bananas)
- Dried fruit (e.g., raisins, apricots, apple rings, mango, peaches)
- Yogurt
- Yogurt drinks
- Toasted nuts (e.g., cashews, peanuts, almonds, brazils)
- Whole-grain breakfast cereal with milk
- Plain popcorn
- Rice cakes
- Fresh, cut vegetables (e.g., carrots, celery, peppers, cucumbers)

- Encourage children to drink water (or diluted fruit juice, if necessary) instead of sugary drinks.

- Don't insist that they must eat everything on the plate; encourage them to try everything and to stop when they are full.

- If you need further advice, consult a qualified nutritionist or registered dietitian.

How Can I Avoid Mealtimes Becoming a Battleground?

Changing children's eating habits is not easy and requires commitment, resolution, and persistence. The sooner you do something about the problem, the better. Provide nutritious meals for everyone; remember not to serve overweight children anything different from the rest of the family. If they refuse certain foods or insist on eating something else, explain that you expect them to try it. Do not give in to unreasonable demands; be resolute and stand firm. If they are hungry, give them only healthy food (fruit, vegetables, grains, nuts), not an extra burger or bowl of ice cream. Keep offering those foods they normally refuse, and encourage them to try new things. The more you "give in" to children's demands for less-healthy food, the harder and longer it will take to establish healthy eating habits. Remember, children can be very controlling and manipulative about food. It may be hard initially, but the eventual rewards will be great.

Should Children Lose Weight for Sports?

Children may feel pressured to lose weight to improve their performance in sports. A lower body-fat percentage can improve running speed, jumping ability, and performance in most sports. However, children should not be encouraged to attain a lower body fat or weight through dieting or excessive exercise, as this can affect their growth and development. They may fail to get all the nutrients they need, causing their health and—ironically—their performance to suffer. Unfortunately, children are often influenced by the successes of thinner teammates or by the remarks of a well-meaning coach.

So what should you do? Children who are a healthy weight for their build should not be encouraged to lose weight. If they are unhappy about

Weight Issues

Many overweight children have low confidence and low self-esteem. Help children develop confidence by praising them for every accomplishment, giving them plenty of opportunities for responsibility, and encouraging them to try new skills (e.g., learning to skate or ride a bike) that foster independence and success.

Let children know that they are loved; give them plenty of one-on-one time and physical affection. Let them know that your love for them is not conditional on their losing weight, and never suggest that you would love them more if they were to lose weight.

their weight, the problem may be one of poor self-esteem or being ill matched to their sport (see Chapter 12). For example, children with a naturally large build are not generally well matched to sports requiring a thin physique, such as long-distance running, ballet, or gymnastics.

If you feel that your children have a genuine weight problem and that losing weight would benefit their performance, health, and self-esteem, follow the advice in this chapter and consult with a registered nutritionist or dietitian. Usually an increase in their daily activity level and training intensity, together with a healthier diet, is all that is needed. Allow plenty of time–months rather than weeks–for fat loss. Under professional guidance, children should lose no more than three to five pounds per month, depending on their age and weight. Weight-loss goals must be realistic and achievable for their build and degree of maturity. They should reach this goal at least three or four weeks before competition. This will allow them to compete at their best. You should discourage strict dieting, diuretics, excessive exercise, and use of saunas as weight-loss methods as they can be very dangerous for growing children. In the short term, these methods could result in an excessive loss of water, low muscle glycogen stores, fatigue, and poor performance. Long term, they could lead to yo-yo dieting, eating disorders, poor health, and impaired development.

How Can I Discourage Television Viewing?

- Be selective about what children watch on television. Let them help you plan exactly what they will watch in advance, and agree upon a defined time period. Once the time period is up, switch off the television, no matter how much they protest!

- Do not place a TV in children's bedrooms.

- Schedule alternative, preferably physically active, pastimes in place of television viewing. If you can keep kids busy with other activities, they won't have much time left for sitting in front of the television.

- Let the number of hours they have exercised equal the number of hours they are allowed to watch television. If they have done an hour's physical activity during the day, you could allocate an hour's television watching.

- Discourage eating meals or snacks while watching television. Because their mind will be on the television and not on the food, they won't notice when they are full or no longer hungry.

CHAPTER 10

Underweight Kids and Fussy Eaters

Some children have small appetites and seem to eat very little, causing enormous worry to their parents. Are they growing properly? Why don't they eat like their friends? Why are they fussy eaters? Trying to feed a fussy eater can be a very frustrating experience that tests a parent's patience and resolve to the limit.

Some children are underweight despite eating normal meals. They struggle to eat enough food to keep their weight up. Active kids who play a lot of sports may burn so much energy that it becomes a problem of how to feed them enough to meet their energy needs. This chapter explores the reasons why some children are underweight, and offers advice on how to encourage a fussy eater to eat normally. It also gives tips on how active children can maintain or gain weight.

Thin or Underweight?

If you are concerned about a child's weight, it's important to work out whether they are clinically underweight or whether they are a thin, yet otherwise perfectly healthy, child. You can reassure yourself that a child is growing normally by asking your doctor to check their height and weight on a standard child growth chart. This will let you know whether their weight is appropriate for their height. If their height is moving parallel to one of the percentile lines and their weight is also moving along in a parallel path, albeit at a slightly lower percentile, they are probably fine. However, if their height or weight has fallen off their usual percentile there may be cause for concern. It may be due to recent illness, but your doctor will be able to check for any underlying medical condition.

Many underweight children have a naturally very lean build. You can ascertain this by looking at their ankle, knee, and wrist joints, and at the width of their shoulders, waist, and hips. A child with small joints and dimensions, who generally eats well, is probably fine.

Why Are Some Children Thin?

There are lots of factors that influence children's weight, shape, and size, but the key ones responsible for a slim build are the following:

- Heredity
- Undereating

HEREDITY

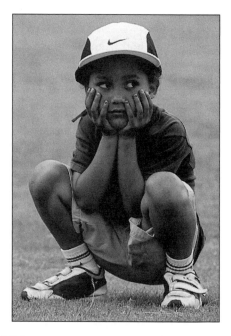

Children inherit their build and basic body shape from their parents (see Chapter 9, "Overweight kids"). You'll notice that children with a thin build have a parent, or sometimes a grandparent, with a similar build. Compare the basic body shapes of parents and their children and you will no doubt see a remarkable resemblance. Thin-built people have strong ectomorphic characteristics—that is, narrow shoulders and hips, long lean limbs, and little body fat. Those narrow joints and slender proportions are inherited and will remain unaffected by what children eat. No amount of food will alter their basic proportions; it will only alter the amount of fat they store. If a thin-built child eats extra calories over and above their needs, they will lay down extra fat—not muscle! Clearly, this is disadvantageous for health or sports. What is needed is a healthy diet that gives children plenty of energy, while supporting muscle growth and good health.

UNDEREATING

Children who consistently fail to eat enough to meet their energy needs will burn energy from their fat stores and muscle tissue. They may therefore end up carrying very little body fat and will have small muscles.

Do your kids eat very little at mealtimes? Many young children have poor appetites, which means they become full after eating relatively little food. See the next section for some practical suggestions on how to feed children with a poor appetite.

Are they fussy eaters? Children often become fussy about food between the ages of one and four years. Choosing and refusing food is one way of asserting their independence. But fussy eating can persist for years, and the longer it is allowed to continue the more difficult it is to get children to accept previously rejected foods. The danger is that fussy eaters could end up failing to consume enough calories and essential nutrients to support peak health and performance. Again, see below for some tips on dealing with fussy eaters.

Do they appear to eat plenty of food but find it a struggle to gain weight? Despite an apparently healthy eating pattern, some children may not be eating enough to meet their high energy needs. They may have a faster than average metabolism, which means they burn calories more quickly to keep up their weight and essential functions such as heart beat, brain function, and digestion. Most children aged seven to ten years need 1,740–1,970 calories; children aged eleven to fourteen years need 1,845–2,220 calories. However, if they play a lot of sports and exercise regularly, they may need considerably more—as many as 3,000 calories a day (see Chapter 7, "Eating for Action"), and that can be quite hard to achieve. The section "Feeding Very Active Children" on page 98 and the box "Snacks for Weight Gain" on page 100 give tips for increasing children's calorie intake.

Feeding Children with Small Appetites

It can be very frustrating trying to feed children who refuse to eat proper meals. You are probably concerned that they're getting too few calories, becoming malnourished, and becoming more vulnerable to illness and infection. The first thing to remember is that children do not voluntarily starve themselves; they are programmed for survival! As long as there is food available, children will make sure they get enough. Second, some children are

very good at using food to wind up their parents. The more firmly they refuse to finish their plate at mealtimes, the more attention they get. They
know that food refusal results in attention (albeit unfavorable), and so a vi-
cious cycle sets up.

So how do you know whether kids are eating enough? Think carefully
about their total daily intake—it may add up to more than you realize. Do
they have snacks between meals? Do they have lots of sugary drinks?
Snacks and beverages can amount to a large proportion of children's daily
food intake. When children consistently refuse meals, many parents are only
too pleased for their child to eat something (even if it's a cookie) rather than
nothing. So it's tempting to give in to demands for snacks.

Now, snacks are not necessarily a bad thing, provided they supply nutrients in proportion to their energy content. But if children are filling up on
cookies, soft drinks, and chips, they won't be getting the vitamins, minerals,
and fiber they need. They will be satisfying their hunger with "empty" calories and have little appetite left for nutritious food at mealtimes.

What's the solution? You need to train children to eat proper meals and
nutritious food. Give them no more than two snacks a day—the first between
breakfast and lunch and the second between lunch and dinner. There should
be no extra snacks if they refuse their meal. Suitable snacks could be fresh
fruit (such as sliced apples, bananas, grapes, or kiwi fruit), cheese, whole-
grain crackers, small sandwiches on whole-grain bread, or a container of yogurt. No matter how much they protest or request unhealthy snacks, stand
firm and do not give them any other food. It will be tough at first—no parent
wants to "starve" their child—but after a week or so they will soon get the
message that the best thing to do at mealtimes is to eat.

Feeding Fussy Eaters

Fussy eating is not just confined to the toddler years. Picky eating habits
often persist for many years, and if they are left unchecked, children do not
just "grow out of them." The earlier you tackle the issue, the better. With
older children it just takes more perseverance. Children are entitled to dislike certain foods, but some children take this to extremes and are frustrat-
ingly fussy. It's not necessary to insist that they clear their plate, but you need
to persuade them that food is enjoyable and fun. Here are some tips to help
you cope with fussy eaters:

- Allow children to help with shopping and meal preparation. This will increase their interest in the food, and they will be more likely to eat the meal if they have been involved in making it.

- Encourage the whole family to eat together whenever possible, and always turn off the television at mealtimes.

- Serve children the same food as the rest of the family.

- Serve small portions (even if they seem ridiculously tiny to you). It's better that they eat a small amount of everything than nothing at all. A big pile of food on the plate can be off-putting for young children.

- Do not discuss eating behavior, food, or family issues at mealtimes. Try to achieve a relaxed atmosphere.

- If they refuse certain foods, explain that you expect them to try it and do not offer an alternative.

- Serve a new food with a food they like.

- Don't keep on telling them to eat up. Children will react to your concern by eating even less and even more slowly.

- Unpopular vegetables can often be disguised—for example, in soup, casseroles, or pasta sauce.

- If kids dislike a particular vegetable, say, Brussels sprouts, serve a similar vegetable, say, broccoli (which is also from the brassica family) or kale (which is also a green, leafy vegetable), which will provide similar nutrients.

- If a food is rejected, it doesn't mean they will never eat it. Keep reintroducing those foods they reject, say, once a week, and don't give up after two or three tries. Remember, it takes up to eight to ten attempts to get a child to eat a new food.

- Allow them to select their own food, but from within a limited choice (e.g., ask, "Would you like broccoli or carrots?" rather than "Would you like vegetables?").

- Try not to fuss if they reject a food or refuse to eat.

- Set a sensible time limit (say, thirty minutes), after which you take away any uneaten food without a fuss.
- If they don't eat their meal, do not give extra food or snacks between meals (see "Feeding Children with Small Appetites," above).
- If they are hungry, offer only nutritious food, not a pastry or chocolate bar.

Hints on Feeding Underweight Children

- Don't fall into the trap of giving in to demands for cookies and chips in the belief that "they need all the calories they can get." Eating these foods between meals will simply take away children's appetites for more nutritious foods at mealtimes, and perpetuate their taste for salty, sugary processed foods.

- If they refuse to eat their meal after the allocated time, remove it without fuss and do not offer any other food (except, perhaps, reheated leftovers from the refused meal) until the next mealtime. Be consistent and rest assured that they won't become malnourished right away. This process won't be easy, but they will soon realize that they only get food at mealtimes.

- Do not fill them up with cookies or sweets after mealtimes. If they are still hungry, offer only nutritious foods, such as fruit, cheese, yogurt, or nuts.

Feeding Very Active Children

For children who struggle to keep up their weight or to put on weight, because they burn a lot of energy in sports, try offering more frequent meals and snacks—six or seven times a day. In fact, snacks are an important part of children's diets. Children have a limited capacity for food, which means they cannot meet their energy demands for growth and activity from three meals only.

The solution is to add on three or four snacks a day, and also to make the energy and nutrient content of the food more concentrated. To gain weight, children need to consume more calories than they use for growth and exercise.

Don't encourage children to reduce the amount of activity or sports they engage in. Exercise offers so many benefits, helping to strengthen their muscles and increase their fitness (see "Strength Training for Children" on the next page).

Here are some suggestions for how to increase the energy intake of children:

- Serve bigger portions, particularly of pasta, potatoes, rice, cereals, dairy products, and protein-rich foods.

- Provide three to four nutritious energy-giving snacks between meals—see box titled "Snacks for Weight Gain" on the next page for suggestions.

- Include nutritious beverages, e.g., milk, homemade milkshakes, yogurt drinks, fruit smoothies, and fruit juice.

- Sprinkle grated cheese on vegetables, soups, potatoes, pasta dishes, and casseroles.

- Add dried fruit to breakfast cereals, hot cereal, and yogurt.

- Spread bread, toast, or crackers with peanut butter or almond butter.

- Serve vegetables and main courses with a sauce, such as cheese sauce.

- Avoid filling your child up on heavy desserts, cookies, and cakes; these supply calories but few essential nutrients (and are usually loaded with saturated or hydrogenated fat).

- Try milk-based or yogurt-based desserts (e.g., rice pudding, banana custard, fruit crumble with yogurt, fruit salad with yogurt or custard, bread pudding, fruit pancakes).

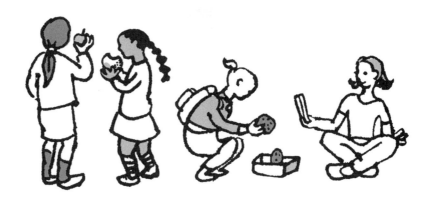

Strength Training for Children[15]

A strength-training or weight-training program designed to improve total fitness will improve children's strength, reduce their risk of sports injuries, and improve their athletic performance. Contrary to the belief that strength training can damage kids' growth cartilage or stunt their growth, recent studies suggest that it can actually make bones stronger. In fact, there are no reported cases of bone damage in relation to strength training. Children who strength train tend to feel better about themselves as they get stronger, and to have higher self-esteem. But strength training is not the same as power lifting, weight lifting, or bodybuilding, none of which are recommended for children under eighteen years old.

Bulking up should not be a goal of a strength-training program. Children and teenagers should tone their muscles using a light weight (or using their

Snacks for Weight Gain

- Nuts—peanuts, almonds, cashews, brazils, pistachios
- Dried fruit—raisins, apple rings, apricots, dates
- Sandwiches on whole-grain bread with cheese, chicken, ham, tuna, peanut butter, or banana
- Yogurt and cottage cheese
- Milk, milkshakes, yogurt drinks
- Breakfast cereal or oatmeal with milk and dried fruit
- Cheese—slices, cubes, or novelty cheese snacks
- Cheese on toast
- Scones, fruit muffins (but if they're not homemade, check the label carefully for hydrogenated fats)
- Small pancakes
- English muffins, rolls, or bagels
- Cereal bars, breakfast bars (make sure they contain no hydrogenated fat), or energy bars
- Whole-grain bread or toast spread with jam or honey

body weight) and a high number of repetitions, rather than lifting heavy weights. Only after they have passed puberty should children consider adding muscle bulk. Younger children should begin with body-weight exercises such as push-ups and sit-ups. More experienced trainees may use free weights and machines.

Sports scientists say that a well-designed strength-training program can bring many fitness benefits for children and can complement an existing training program. Indeed, the American Academy of Pediatrics Committee on Sports Medicine endorses strength training. Here are some guidelines:

- Children should be properly supervised during training sessions.
- They should use an age-appropriate routine (adult routines are not suitable)–typically thirty-second intervals with breaks in-between, with thorough warm-up and cool-down periods.
- Ensure that the exercises are performed using proper form and technique.
- Children should start with a relatively light weight and a high number of repetitions.
- No heavy lifts should be included.
- The program should form part of a total fitness program.
- The sessions should be varied and fun.

Note: Children should undergo a complete medical examination before beginning a strength-training program.

CHAPTER 11

Eating at School

Are you happy about what your children eat for lunch at school? How can you be sure they are getting a balanced meal that sets them up for the afternoon? How can you influence what they choose to eat at school?

A healthy midday meal helps children to concentrate and participate more fully in class. It will provide them with sustained energy to fuel their muscles and their brains. On the other hand, eating the wrong foods will reduce their physical and mental performance.

The healthiest option for eating at school is usually a home-packed lunch. At least then you have control over what children eat for lunch, and this can make a real difference to their health. It's easy to get stuck in a rut, but altering the contents of kids' lunchbox throughout the week will ensure that they get plenty of variety in their diet, and this can be a great way of introducing them to new foods. This chapter gives you some guidelines on putting together a perfectly balanced lunch and plenty of ideas to make lunches inspiring. It also offers suggestions for interesting sandwiches and healthy treats.

For children who eat a school lunch, there is less scope for influencing what they eat. This chapter lists recommended nutritional guidelines for school meals and includes some hints on encouraging your child to make the best choices.

What are the best foods to eat after school? Whether they play sports or do homework after school, children need nutritious foods to bridge the gap between school and dinner. This chapter will give you lots of ideas for healthy snacks.

What Are Children Eating at School?[16]

- Children's favorite items on the school menu are pizza and burgers, according to a survey by school meal caterers.

- One in three children buys candy, chocolate, soft drinks, chips, or other unhealthy snacks on the way to and from school.

- Children eat fries for lunch between two and three times a week.

Packing a Healthy Lunch

What you put in children's lunchboxes is critical for balancing their day's nutritional intake. Lunch should supply approximately one-third of a child's daily energy needs, as well as one-third of their protein, carbohydrate, fiber, vitamin, and mineral needs. But getting children to eat a nutritious lunch at school is not always easy. The food you provide has got to look exciting, taste good, and be easy to eat. You don't want them returning their lunchbox contents uneaten or, worse, disposing of it in the garbage can at school. It's easy to fall into the trap of filling kids' lunchboxes with treats, chips, and chocolate bars to make sure that "they at least eat something at school." The problem is that these types of food will quickly become the focus of the meal, and other foods will be ignored.

There's also peer pressure for kids to eat the same kind of foods as their friends are eating. Do they insist on having a bag of chips every day to be like their friends? Again, chips and savory snacks can displace healthier foods in the lunchbox, and chip eating can become the norm. Save such food for occasional treats.

Here is a guide to making up a balanced lunchbox menu, based on the Food Pyramid in Chapter 2.

BALANCING THE PERFECT LUNCHBOX

- A drink (six to eight fluid ounces)

- One or two portions of fresh or dried fruit

- One portion of salad or vegetables (e.g., in a sandwich filling, or as cut-up vegetables)

- Two to three portions from the grains group (e.g., either two or three slices of bread, a bagel, four to six crackers, a small tub of pasta, or a cereal bar)

- One portion from the dairy group (e.g., cheese, yogurt, cottage cheese, or milk)

- One portion from the protein-rich food group (e.g., meat, fish, dairy, nuts, beans)

Beverages

A lunchtime beverage will keep children well hydrated and thereby help them avoid flagging energy levels in the afternoon. Even mild dehydration can causes headaches, fatigue, and poor concentration. Remember, children need six to eight glasses of fluid a day (see Chapter 8, "Drinking for Action"). Drinking plenty of fluid is also important to help their kidneys, brain, and digestive system work properly.

Lunchtime Beverages

BEST CHOICES	LESS SUITABLE
Water	Soft drinks (contain too much sugar and too many artificial additives)
Milk or milkshake (keep chilled in a thermos)	Artificially flavored/colored fruit drinks and fruit punches (contain too much sugar and too many artificial additives)
Fruit juice (diluted one part juice, two parts water)	Sugar-free and "diet" drinks (contain artificial sweeteners and additives)

Fruit and Vegetables

A piece of fresh fruit in children's lunchboxes will help make up the daily goal of the two portions suggested in the Food Pyramid (see Chapter 2). All types of fruit and vegetables—including dried and canned varieties—supply vitamins, minerals, and phytochemicals (see Chapter 6, "Vitamins and Minerals"). Fruits that are easy to eat or prepare are best (see the box on the next page). If a whole piece of fruit is unappealing, chop it into pieces or supply a knife (e.g., for apples) or spoon (e.g., for kiwi fruit) to make it easier for them to eat. When my six-year-old first took a kiwi fruit with a small

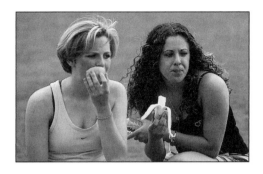

knife and spoon to school, her friends were so intrigued they requested one too! Small easy-open cans of fruit in juice and small cartons of fruit purée are also ideal for lunchboxes—look out for them in your supermarket.

Small boxes and bags of dried fruit are also good choices. They are fun to eat and supply good amounts of fiber and various vitamins. My four-year-old daughter adores dried mango pieces in her lunchbox. Dried mango and apricots are rich in beta-carotene and iron. The downside, though, is that they tend to stick to the teeth, like sweets, so encourage children to brush their teeth afterwards or to follow with an apple or piece of cheese (this reduces the acidity and helps remineralize the tooth enamel).

Try packing carrot, pepper, celery, or cucumber sticks (wrapped in plastic wrap or in a small zip-lock bag) or putting salad vegetables (e.g., cherry tomatoes, tomatoes, cucumbers) in sandwiches.

BEST FRUIT CHOICES

Apples, pears

Oranges, mandarins, tangerines

Bananas

Grapes

Kiwi fruit (children can cut them in half and scoop out the flesh with a spoon)

Cherries

Small container of strawberries, blueberries, or raspberries

Peaches, nectarines

Small boxes of raisins

Small bags of apricots, mango, pineapple, raisins, dried-fruit mixtures

Easy-open cans or long-life cartons of fruit in juice

Cartons of fruit purée

BEST VEGETABLE CHOICES

Sticks of carrots, cucumber, peppers

Baby corn

Tomato, cucumber, or lettuce in a sandwich filling

Cherry tomatoes

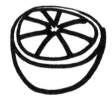

Sandwiches and Fillers

Starchy carbohydrates should supply at least half of the calories in the lunchbox. This translates to about two slices of bread, a bagel, or a small tub of pasta or rice. Sandwiches and bagels are a popular and easy choice. Vary kids' usual sandwiches by providing different types of bread. Try mini pita pockets, tortilla wraps (cut into short lengths), a bagel, or an English muffin. Try making sandwiches with different types of bread, such as walnut bread, raisin or fruit bread, seeded bread, or cheese and herb bread.

The filling should include a protein-rich food (such as cheese, chicken, ham, turkey, peanut butter, tuna, or hummus) and, ideally, a salad vegetable (such as cucumber or tomato). Don't use jam, honey, or chocolate-spread fillings too often as they contain mostly sugar and no protein. Save them as treats, and instead provide some extra cheese or yogurt.

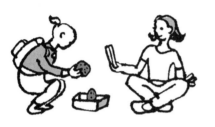

Fed up with sandwiches? Pasta and rice salads can be jazzed up with chopped vegetables, nuts, dried fruit, beans, chopped chicken, or tuna (see recipes on pages 137, 144, 161).

The box below gives ideas for sandwiches and healthy sandwich fillings.

BREADS/GRAINS	SANDWICH FILLINGS
Whole-grain, malted grain, or wheat-germ bread	Lean ham and tomato
Whole-grain rolls	Peanut butter with grated cheese
Mini pita bread	Peanut butter with banana or fruit spread
English muffin	Hummus and tomato
Mini bagel	Low-fat cream cheese with tuna
Tortilla wrap	Mozzarella and tomato
Bread sticks	Egg salad, chicken salad, or tuna salad
Whole-grain crackers	Banana and honey
Potato salad	Turkey slices with cranberry sauce
Pasta or rice salad	Avocado slices and chicken
	Hummus and grated carrot
	Cottage cheese and pineapple
	Salmon and cucumber
	Chopped chicken and coleslaw

Dairy Products

Include one dairy food in the lunchbox (see the box below for ideas). This is easier to do nowadays, with the availability of lunchbox-size coolers that will keep perishable foods at refrigerated temperatures for hours. Soy alternatives (e.g., soy cheese, soy yogurt, soy milk, and soy milkshakes) are also available if your children cannot tolerate dairy products. Both dairy and soy products supply protein as well as valuable calcium. Be sure to check the label of yogurts for artificial sweeteners, colors, and flavorings, and try to keep these to a minimum. In general, organic varieties and "toddler" varieties of these foods are best as they don't contain additives. Yogurt pouches and tubes are great for eating on the go as they don't require a spoon.

Lunchbox Dairy Products

- Cheese in the sandwich filling
- Chunks or slices of cheese
- Novelty cheese product (e.g., individual cheddar portions, cheese strips, or string cheese)
- Carton or tube of yogurt
- Milk
- Milkshake
- Yogurt drink
- Carton of custard

Treats

Treats, such as chocolate-coated bars, candy, chips, and cookies, should not be included every day! They are loaded with fat and sugar and provide very little nutritional value. These foods tend to cling to the teeth (yes, even savory snacks), so unless children brush their teeth after lunch, these snacks can increase the chances of developing tooth decay.

A weekly treat is fine, but encourage children to brush their teeth or eat a small piece of cheese afterward; this helps counteract some of the damaging effects of sugar. My six-year-old daughter takes a fun travel toothbrush in her lunchbox, much to the initial amusement of her friends, who now join in the toothbrushing routine, too!

A lot of parents provide a treat as a way of saying "I'm thinking about you and I care for you." But you can say this in other ways. Why not pop in a little note that says "I love you" or a favorite cartoon, picture, or joke? My daughter eagerly anticipates the surprise note or joke I put in her lunchbox, passes it around to her friends, and then collects the jokes in a special folder. At least she has a lasting reminder of lunchbox treats that don't damage her teeth!

The box below gives ideas for healthier treats:

Healthy Lunchbox Treats

- Fruit muffin or teacake

- Mini pancake

- Cereal bar or breakfast bar

- Scone

- Breadsticks

- Rice cakes

- Plain popcorn

- Plain reduced-fat chips

- Homemade cakes and muffins (see recipes on pages 194–199)

- Small bags of dried fruit (e.g., raisins, mango, apricots, dates, pineapple)

What's in School Meals?

The United States hasn't established government-mandated nutritional guidelines for school lunches overall. However, if a school wants to participate in the National School Lunch Program, a federally subsidized meal program for low-income schoolchildren, the lunches offered must meet the recommendations of the Dietary Guidelines for Americans, as established by the U.S. government. In general, these are as follows:[17]

- No more than 30 percent of an individual's calories should come from fat, and less than 10 percent should come from saturated fat.

- School lunches must provide one-third of the Recommended Dietary Allowances for protein, vitamin A, vitamin C, iron, calcium, and calories.

Twelve Lunchbox Ideas

1. Chicken and tomato sandwich on whole-grain bread, a container of yogurt, carrot sticks, a mandarin orange, and a drink of orange juice (diluted).

2. Peanut butter and cucumber sandwich, a slice of cheese, strawberries, yogurt in a tube, and a bottle of water.

3. Slice of homemade pizza, strips of peppers, cherry tomatoes, an apple, yogurt drink, and a bottle of water.

4. Pasta salad with tuna, peppers, and mushrooms, container of yogurt, small bag of dried apricots, and an apple juice (diluted).

5. Tortilla wrap filled with cooked turkey and coleslaw, a small easy-open can of fruit in juice, and a carton of milk.

6. Mini bagel filled with cream cheese and sliced banana, a small bunch of grapes, a container of yogurt, and a bottle of water.

7. Rice salad with cooked chicken, peas, and corn; a pear; a container of chocolate milk; and a bottle of water.

8. Cooked soy sausage, egg-salad sandwich on whole-grain bread, a handful of nuts (e.g., cashews or peanuts), tangerines, fruit juice (diluted).

9. Whole-grain crackers, hummus dip, cubes of cheese, grapes, a container of yogurt, and a bottle of water.

10. Mini pita filled with canned salmon, lettuce, and tomato; cherries; mini box of raisins; a yogurt drink; and a bottle of water.

11. Peanut butter sandwich on whole-grain bread, tub of mixed-bean salad, a peach, a carton of custard, and an orange juice (diluted).

12. Whole-grain roll filled with tuna, corn, and mayonnaise; carrot sticks; cheese slice; small bag of dried fruit (e.g., mango, pineapple); and a bottle of water.

What Should I Encourage Children to Eat for School Lunch?

If your child eats a school lunch, here are a few guidelines to discuss with him or her about how to make healthier choices:

	HEALTHIER OPTIONS	AVOID
Main course	Chicken or fish dishes (but not fried)	Hamburgers, hot dogs
	Baked beans or bean casseroles	Sausages
	Vegetable, chicken, or lentil soup	Chicken nuggets, fried chicken
	Pizza	Meat pies
	Pasta dishes with tomato or vegetable-based sauces	Batter-fried fish
	Chicken, turkey, or vegetable stews	Pasta dishes with creamy or oily sauces
		Anything that appears excessively oily (e.g., chili, tacos, some pizzas)
Accompaniments	Baked potatoes filled with tuna, steamed veggies, cheese, or coleslaw	French fries
Vegetables	Vegetable casseroles	
	Potatoes—boiled, mashed, or baked	
	At least one portion of vegetables or salad	
Dessert	Fresh fruit (at least three times a week)	Cookies
	Fruit-based desserts (e.g. fruit crumble, banana custard)	Cakes
		Sweet rolls, cinnamon buns, pastries
	Yogurt pudding	Fried fruit or custard pies
	Milk-based pudding (e.g., rice pudding)	
Beverages	Water	Soft drinks
	Fruit juice	Fruit drinks, fruit punch
	Milk	Sugar-free and diet drinks

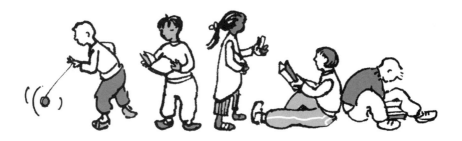

What Can I Give Children after School?

Children always seem to be starving when they come home from school, so that is a good time to offer a healthy snack. It will bridge the gap between lunch and dinner, and if they are playing a sport or playing active games with their friends, it will fuel their muscles and help their performance (see Chapter 7, "Food for Action").

Bread, toast, crackers, and fruit are good choices as they are high in carbohydrate and also provide a range of vitamins and minerals. Balance the snack with a glass of milk, a handful of nuts or seeds, a container of yogurt, or a piece of cheese. These foods all provide protein and calcium and when combined with a carbohydrate food give a more sustained release of energy.

Don't give in to demands for sweets, cookies, and candy. It's easy to think that kids "deserve" a treat after school, but once they get into the habit of eating well, they will be equally happy with healthy foods. My children and their friends delight in a plate of crackers, cheese, and apple slices. Remember, sweets and cookies provide only empty calories and will not provide lasting energy. They are high-GI foods (see Chapter 4), imparting a rapid rise in blood sugar followed by a rapid fall. The result? Flagging energy levels,

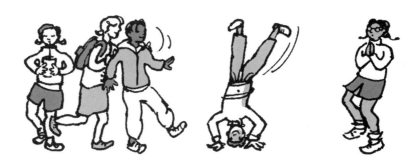

poor concentration, and hunger. If your children play a sport, they need a snack that will help them maintain their energy and keep them from tiring before the end of the game or practice session. Even if they will be doing homework or a similar sedentary activity, they need a snack that will maintain concentration and stave off hunger.

The box below gives some ideas for after-school snacks.

After-School Snacks

Accompany with a drink of water or diluted fruit juice (one part juice to one part water).

- A piece of fresh fruit and a glass of milk
- Whole-grain toast and hummus with a handful of nuts
- Cereal bar, breakfast bar, or energy bar
- A container of yogurt and a small bag of dried fruit
- A bowl of breakfast cereal with milk
- Mini pancake or scone and cottage cheese
- Crackers with cheese
- Homemade fruit muffins or cakes (see recipes on pages 194–199)
- Fruit smoothies
- Peanut butter sandwich

CHAPTER 12

Eating Disorders

It is not unusual for young teenagers to become more body conscious, but if they become preoccupied with their weight and develop negative thoughts about their appearance, this could signal the beginning of an eating disorder. Eating disorders are increasingly common among children and teenagers, especially girls. Surveys have revealed that an alarming number of normal-weight girls perceive themselves as overweight and want to lose weight. Ninety percent of children and teenagers with eating disorders are girls.

This chapter will help you decide whether the teenager you know may have an eating disorder. It describes the warning signs and offers some explanation as to why some young girls—and athletes in particular—develop eating disorders. It gives suggestions for how to support children with eating disorders and discusses how to prevent them.

What Are Eating Disorders?

Generally, eating disorders involve negative, self-critical thoughts and feelings about appearance and food. Sufferers are preoccupied with food and their weight. Food may be seen as a penalty for perceived failure or as a source of comfort. By controlling their food intake, sufferers believe that they are in control of one particular situation. A person with anorexia literally starves her- or himself thin, eating very little or no food. Bulimia is a condition of bingeing and purging, whereby a person secretly eats vast quantities of food and then either regurgitates it by making herself vomit or misuses laxatives to cause the food to pass through the body before nutrients and calories have been absorbed.

> • In a survey of twelve- to fourteen-year-old girls, 12 percent admitted to binge eating, and 7 percent said they used self-induced vomiting to lose weight (Source: Princess Margaret Hospital, Toronto).
>
> • Eating-disorder clinics report that girls as young as eight are being admitted for the treatment of eating disorders.
>
> • Many five-year-old girls are already concerned with their shape and about being fat (Source: Women's Hospital, Boston).
>
> • Seventy percent of normal-weight girls aged eleven to eighteen years thought they were too fat (Source: Institute of Psychiatry).
>
> • Up to 62 percent of girls involved in certain sports, such as gymnastics and endurance running, have abnormal eating behavior.[18]

What Are the Causes of Eating Disorders?

There is no single cause; rather, a whole series of circumstances or pressures make a person develop an eating disorder. It may be triggered by a serious life event, such as a divorce, illness, or death in the family, or in some cases by an insignificant event, such as a comment made about the person's weight. But there are nearly always other underlying factors involved. These can include family problems, relationships, low self-esteem, problems at school, and a fear of failure. There may also be an intense desire for athletic success and a belief that weight loss will allow the person to perform better in competition.

It is worth remembering that adolescence is a difficult time for young girls, as they learn to adjust to their changing body shape as well as to the responsibilities of growing up. They also need to deal with the pressures of school and other adolescent stresses, such as their developing sexuality and their identity as young women.

Why Are Eating Disorders Common among Young Athletes?

Eating disorders are more common among teenagers involved in sports in which a low body weight or low body-fat percentage is thought to be advantageous: endurance running, figure skating, gymnastics, and dancing. In susceptible children, the demands of certain sports or the requests made by coaches to lose weight may trigger an eating disorder. For example, in their determination to improve their performance and achieve competitive success, some children mistakenly believe that thinness will lead to greater success in their sport. They then become obsessed with weight loss. They may identify with elite athletes in their particular sport who are inherently slim—natural ectomorphs (see Chapter 9)—and model themselves on their thin physiques. Of course, many other factors besides body weight are involved in achieving success, including training, natural ability, and mental preparation. Proper nutrition is essential for training, so if athletes cut down on their calorie intake, their performance will suffer. Misguided weight-loss attempts are counterproductive; instead of providing the hoped-for success in their sport, they produce a negative effect on an athlete's performance.

Parents and Food

Do you have a healthy attitude toward food? Do you worry about your own weight and shape? Have you regularly dieted or tried to watch your weight? Some experts believe that children's attitudes toward food and their body image may be passed down from their parents. Children learn by example. If children see their mothers shunning snack foods or counting calories, they are likely to do the same. A mother's excessive worry about food may rub off on her daughter or son.

- A study involving one hundred young children concluded that dieting parents or those who are overanxious about food may be to blame for their children's unhealthy attitudes toward eating and their bodies (Source: Glasgow University).

- Mothers who dislike body fat are communicating that attitude to their children (Source: St Mary's Hospital, London).

- Overprotective, uncommunicative parents are more likely to raise children who will develop an eating disorder (Source: Manchester University).

Children with a personality predisposed to eating disorders may be attracted to certain sports, such as endurance running, because they see it as another method of weight loss. They may compete at events, but their main motivation for running remains the pursuit of slimness.

How Do I Know If a Child Has an Eating Disorder?

Look at the lists of warning signs for anorexia nervosa and bulimia nervosa in the box below. These will help you to recognize potential problems in your children. The presence of only one or two signs does not necessarily mean that they have an eating disorder. It is important to seek advice from an appropriate health-care professional for a proper diagnosis and the right kind of help.

How Will an Eating Disorder Affect a Child's Health and Performance?

Eating too little over a period of time can be physically and emotionally harmful. Initially, anorexic athletes appear to have endless energy and are capable of pushing themselves through hard training sessions. But as sufferers lose more weight, their athletic performance drops. They will eventually feel too tired to train as their bodies become too weak. Rather than helping them perform better in sports, eating too little will ultimately cause them to stop exercising altogether.

In girls, menstruation usually stops (or doesn't start in young teens), increasing the risk of brittle bones. They may suffer repeated injuries and stress fractures and, in the long term, risk premature osteoporosis.

Many athletes with bulimia appear to cope with training, but inside they feel out of control and worthless. Repeated use of laxatives, diuretics, and vomiting can damage their health. They can develop bad breath, dental erosion and decay, dehydration, and kidney and bowel problems.

Warning Signs for Anorexia Nervosa

- Dramatic loss of weight
- Preoccupation with food, calories, and weight
- Exercising excessively
- Mood swings
- Avoiding social situations where food is served
- Periods stop or have never started
- Feeling fat even when underweight
- Setting unreasonably high standards
- Lying about eating meals and refusing to eat in the company of others

Warning Signs for Bulimia Nervosa

- Extreme weight fluctuations
- Swollen salivary glands
- Irregular periods
- Excessive concern about weight
- Visiting the bathroom during or after meals
- Increasingly self-critical of her body and performance
- Emotional and depressed, mood swings
- Feeling out of control
- Eating large amounts of food followed by strict dieting
- Takes laxatives or diuretics

What Can I Do If I Think a Child Has an Eating Disorder?

If you suspect a child may be worrying too much about their weight or developing an eating disorder, there are a number of things you can do to help. Talk to them and listen to their concerns, but avoid making comments about their appearance. Whatever you say about their appearance may be misinterpreted. Instead, show lots of love and respect. If they deny that they have a problem, keep persevering. Sufferers of eating disorders do their best to keep their condition a secret as long as possible, but often they want help and do not know whom to ask. They may feel embarrassed and their self-esteem may feel threatened, so you must avoid a direct confrontation about their weight loss or eating behavior. Do not present them with "evidence" of their disorder. Instead, let them know that you are there if they need to talk, and offer unconditional support. Don't fight with them about food.

Once a child has admitted to having a problem, encourage them to seek help. You can listen, but don't try to give advice if you are not qualified to do so. The earlier a problem is identified, the shorter the treatment period and the better the chances of successful treatment. There are various resources available for help, including trained counselors from a self-help organization (see Resources) as well as your family doctor, who will be able to refer the child to a psychologist or dietitian specializing in eating disorders.

Preventing Eating Disorders

Your own behavior may help children avoid eating disorders. By focusing on their strengths you will help them build self-esteem. Here are some pointers for fostering a positive body image and preventing eating disorders:

- Support your children for what they are as well as what they do or what they look like.
- Be a healthy example: Avoid making negative comments about your own body (e.g., "I'm fat") in front of children and teenagers.
- Aim for moderation in food and exercise; your children will be more likely to do as you do.
- Teach children to feel good about themselves, regardless of body size or shape.
- Reassure adolescents that the physical changes they are experiencing are normal, and that everyone develops at their own rate.
- Discuss body-image issues as they arise; always give reassurance and emphasize your child's individuality.

- Help your children develop a critical awareness of the images and messages portrayed in the media.

- Never use food as a punishment or reward.

- Emphasize nutrition and enjoyment; look at the health-giving properties of food rather than the calories or fat.

- Do not force your children to eat when they are not hungry; encourage them to listen to their natural appetite cues.

- Do not pressure your children to eat only low-fat "healthy" food, and do not ban fatty foods or sweets. Doing so could have the opposite effect to the one intended.

- Mealtimes should not be stressful.

- Encourage children to enjoy all forms of physical activities and to appreciate that movement is fun. Exercise should not be portrayed as a method of weight loss.

- Parents who follow a weight-loss diet should emphasize that this is not right for a child.

CHAPTER 13

Kids' Menu Plans

Use the following menu plans to help you feed your children the right balance of carbohydrates, protein, fat, vitamins, and minerals. Remember, the emphasis should be on variety and enjoyment. Introduce new foods and flavors at every opportunity. Make healthy snacks easily accessible, and limit the amount of unhealthy food in your household. Encourage your children to drink six to eight glasses of fluid (water, diluted fruit juice, milk) daily, and an additional half cup to a cup of fluid for each hour of exercise (see Chapter 8, "Drinking for Action").

I've included two seven-day menu plans for five- to ten-year-olds and two seven-day menu plans for eleven- to fifteen-year-olds. One of the two plans for each age group is vegetarian. Choose a serving size based on your children's age, appetite, and specific requirements (see Chapter 2, "What Should Active Children Eat?"). All of these menu plans include several recipes I've developed and that have passed the "kid-approved" test. These recipes start in Chapter 14.

Located immediately after the seven-day menu plans are ideas for after-school snacks and lunchbox treats, and for after-sport snacks.

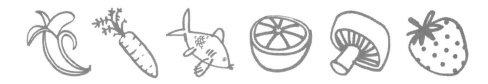

Seven-Day Menu Plan for Five- to Ten-Year-Olds

Monday	Breakfast	Whole-grain cereal with milk Banana
	Lunchbox	Tuna, tomato, and mayonnaise sandwich Small easy-open can of fruit in juice Carton of yogurt Water
	Supper	Chicken Burgers *(see recipe on page 171)* Oven Potato Wedges *(see recipe on page 182)* Baked beans, broccoli Stewed apples and raisins
Tuesday	Breakfast	Whole-grain toast and peanut butter Fresh fruit Milk or yogurt
	Lunchbox	Slice of pizza Carrot, celery, and cucumber crudités A bunch of seedless grapes Cottage cheese or yogurt Orange juice
	Supper	Pasta and Tuna Bake *(see recipe on page 139)* Sliced tomatoes with a little dressing Yogurt and fruit
Wednesday	Breakfast	Oatmeal or cream of wheat made with milk and water A little honey and raisins
	Lunchbox	Pita bread filled with cold chopped chicken and coleslaw Dried apricots Milk
	Supper	Toad-and-Vegetables-in-the-Hole *(see recipe on page 136)* Spring cabbage or broccoli Fresh fruit
Thursday	Breakfast	Banana Smoothie *(see recipe on page 203)*
	Lunchbox	Whole-grain roll filled with lean ham and tomato Piece of fresh fruit Container of custard Bottle of water

Seven-Day Menu Plan for Five- to Ten-Year-Olds (cont'd.)

	Supper	Baked potato filled with baked beans and grated cheese OR filled with scrambled egg and tomato Crunchy Apple Crumble *(see recipe on page 186)*
Friday	Breakfast	Bowl of fresh fruit (e.g., oranges, pineapple, and mango) Carton of fruit yogurt
	Lunchbox	Cheese dip or Hummus *(see recipe on page 193)*, breadsticks Crudités (e.g., carrot, red and green pepper, and celery strips) Small box of raisins Milkshake
	Supper	Chicken Baked in Tomato Sauce *(see recipe on page 131)* Boiled rice, peas Fresh fruit
Saturday	Breakfast	Scrambled egg and whole-grain toast Orange juice
	Lunch	Potato Soup *(see recipe on page 164)* Grated cheese Whole-grain roll Fresh fruit salad *(see recipes on pages 191–192)*
	Supper	Homemade Chicken Nuggets *(see recipe on page 170)* Mighty Root Mash *(see recipe on page 181)* Carrots and peas Baked Rice Pudding *(see recipe on page 187)*
Sunday	Breakfast	Crepes filled with apple purée *(see recipe on page 185)*
	Lunch	Baked potato Grilled chicken Broccoli and carrots Raspberry Fool *(see recipe on page 184)*
	Supper	Cheese and Tomato Pizza *(see recipe on page 179)* with any of the suggested toppings Salad: cherry tomatoes, peppers, grated carrot, cucumber A little salad dressing Fresh fruit

Seven-Day Menu Plan for Ten- to Fifteen-Year-Olds

Monday   Breakfast   Oatmeal or cream of wheat made with milk and water
Raisins

Lunchbox   Bagel with low-fat cream cheese and canned tuna or
salmon
Cherry tomatoes
Carton of yogurt
Piece of fresh fruit
Bottle of water

Supper   Vegetable and Pasta Soup *(see recipe on page 169)*
Whole-grain roll
Banana and Nut Fool *(see recipe on page 190)*

Tuesday   Breakfast   English muffin or bagel with jam or honey
Yogurt or milk

Lunchbox   Small container of pasta salad with tuna
Orange or kiwi fruit
Small bag of nuts and raisins
Fruit juice

Supper   Marvelous Macaroni and Cheese *(see recipe on page 147)*
Broccoli and carrots
Baked Bananas *(see recipe on page 189)*

Wednesday   Breakfast   Whole-grain cereal with milk
Fresh fruit
Whole-grain toast and honey

Lunchbox   Whole-grain roll with turkey and cranberry sauce
Crudités (e.g., cucumber, red and green pepper, and car-
rot strips)
Cheese slice
Piece of fresh fruit
Bottle of water

Supper   Pasta with Corn and Tuna *(see recipe on page 137)*
Brussels sprouts or broccoli
Poached pears

Seven-Day Menu Plan for Ten- to Fifteen-Year-Olds (cont'd.)

Thursday	Breakfast	Mango and Strawberry Smoothie *(see recipe on page 204)*
	Lunchbox	Thermos of tomato or vegetable soup Whole-grain bagel with cheese Small bag of dried apricots Bottle of water
	Supper	Grilled chicken Baked potato Baby corn and sugar snap peas
Friday	Breakfast	Granola with milk or yogurt Strawberries or raspberries
	Lunchbox	Egg-salad sandwich on whole-grain bread Carrot and celery slices Carton of yogurt Banana Muffin *(see recipe on page 195)* Bottle of water
	Supper	Fish Cakes *(see recipe on page 143)* Carrots and peas Banana Bread Pudding *(see recipe on page 188)*
Saturday	Breakfast	Crepes filled with fresh fruit *(see recipe on page 185)*
	Lunch	Butternut Squash Soup *(see recipe on page 167)* Whole-grain roll Fresh fruit salad with frozen yogurt
	Supper	Pasta Turkey Bolognese *(see recipe on page 133)* Broccoli and cauliflower Crunchy Apple Crumble *(see recipe on page 186)*
Sunday	Breakfast	Boiled egg and whole-grain toast Nectarine or pear
	Lunch	Golden Baked Chicken *(see recipe on page 134)* Mashed potatoes and green beans Fresh fruit salad with frozen yogurt or custard
	Supper	Sardines on whole-grain toast Baked beans and coleslaw Yogurt and Fruit Pudding *(see recipe on page 189)*

Seven-Day Vegetarian Menu Plan for Five- to Ten-Year-Olds

Monday

Breakfast — Granola with milk or yogurt
Orange juice

Lunchbox — Spicy Bean Burger *(see recipe on page 172)* wrapped in foil
Small whole-grain bun
Crudités (e.g., carrots, peppers, cucumber)
Piece of fruit
Carton of yogurt
Bottle of water

Supper — Vegetarian Spaghetti Bolognese *(see recipe on page 145)*
Fresh fruit with custard or frozen yogurt

Tuesday

Breakfast — Oatmeal or cream of wheat made with milk, water, honey
Raisins

Lunchbox — Peanut butter and fruit spread sandwich on whole-grain bread
Small bag of dried apricots
String cheese
Orange juice

Supper — Broccoli and Cheese Soup *(see recipe on page 166)*
Whole-grain roll
Baked Bananas with yogurt *(see recipe on page 189)*

Wednesday

Breakfast — Banana Milkshake *(see recipe on page 202)*
Whole-grain toast and peanut butter

Lunchbox — Mini bagel filled with turkey and light cream cheese
Mandarin orange
Carton of custard
Orange juice

Supper — Potato and Cheese Pie *(see recipe on page 158)*
Green beans and carrots
Baked Rice Pudding with fresh fruit *(see recipe on page 187)*

Thursday

Breakfast — Whole-grain cereal with milk
Orange juice

Lunchbox — Hummus dip *(see recipe on page 193)*
Breadsticks or crackers
Crudités (e.g., carrot, red and green pepper, and cucumber strips)

Seven-Day Vegetarian Menu Plan for Five- to Ten-Year-Olds (cont'd.)

		Small carton of applesauce Cottage cheese Bottle of water
	Supper	Spicy Lentil Burgers *(see recipe on page 174)* Baked potato Baked beans and broccoli Fresh fruit salad
Friday	Breakfast	Whole-grain toast and jam or fruit spread Fresh fruit (e.g., apple or strawberries) Milk or yogurt
	Lunchbox	Mini pita with grated cheese and tomato Small bag of nuts (e.g., almonds, cashews, peanuts) Piece of fresh fruit Apple Muffin *(see recipe on page 194)* Bottle of water
	Supper	Marvelous Macaroni and Cheese *(see recipe on page 147)* Cauliflower and broccoli Raspberry Fool *(see recipe on page 184)*
Saturday	Breakfast	Poached egg Tomatoes Whole-grain toast with peanut butter
	Lunch	Carrot Soup *(see recipe on page 168)* with grated cheese Whole-grain roll
	Supper	Butter Bean and Leek Supper *(see recipe on page 154)* New potatoes and carrots Yogurt
Sunday	Breakfast	Crepes filled with fresh fruit *(see recipe on page 185)* Orange juice
	Lunch	Nut Burgers *(see recipe on page 175)* Baked potato Carrots and Brussels sprouts or broccoli Banana Bread Pudding *(see recipe on page 188)*
	Supper	Cheese on whole-grain toast Tomatoes and cucumber Yogurt

Seven-Day Vegetarian Menu Plan for Ten- to Fifteen-Year-Olds

Monday

Breakfast
English muffin or bagel with a slice of cheese
Fresh fruit

Lunchbox
Pasta salad with red kidney beans, sweet peppers, and tomatoes
Carton of yogurt
Small bag of dried fruit
Bottle of water

Supper
Cauliflower covered in cheese
Baked potato and green beans
Baked Bananas *(see recipe on page 189)*

Tuesday

Breakfast
Whole-grain cereal with milk
Raisins or dried apricots

Lunchbox
Whole-grain roll with sliced avocado and tomato
Cheese cubes
Piece of fresh fruit
Container of chocolate milk

Supper
Cheese and Tomato Pizza *(see recipe on page 179)* with any of the suggested toppings
Baked potato
Coleslaw or salad
Fresh fruit

Wednesday

Breakfast
Oatmeal or cream of wheat made with milk and water
Banana

Lunchbox
Thermos of vegetable soup
Whole-grain roll
Small bunch of seedless grapes
Orange juice

Supper
Chickpea and Spinach Pasta *(see recipe on page 149)*
Fresh fruit salad with yogurt or custard

Thursday

Breakfast
Granola mixed with grated apple
Milk or yogurt

Lunchbox
Cooked vegetarian sausage, wrapped in foil
Hummus on a whole-grain bagel
Small bag of nuts (e.g., almonds, cashews, peanuts)

Seven-Day Vegetarian Menu Plan for Ten- to Fifteen-Year-Olds (cont'd.)

		Cottage cheese Bottle of water
	Supper	Bean Burritos *(see recipe on page 152)* Salad or broccoli Stewed pears with raisins and honey
Friday	Breakfast	Energizer *(see recipe on page 205)* Whole-grain toast
	Lunchbox	English muffin with peanut butter and cheese Carrot sticks Carton of yogurt Small bag of dried fruit Fruit juice
	Supper	Vegetable Korma *(see recipe on page 155)* Rice Fresh fruit salad
Saturday	Breakfast	Scrambled egg with mushrooms Whole-grain toast
	Lunch	Spicy Bean Burger *(see recipe on page 172)* Whole-grain bun Salad Fresh fruit
	Supper	Baked potato filled with stir-fried or steamed vegetables Crunchy Apple Crumble (or other fruit variety; *see recipe on page 186)* Custard or yogurt
Sunday	Breakfast	Crepes filled with sliced bananas and honey *(see recipe on page 185)*
	Lunch	Red beans and rice Carrots and broccoli Cherry Clafouti *(see recipe on page 190)*
	Supper	Real Tomato Soup *(see recipe on page 165)* with grated cheese Whole-grain roll Fresh fruit

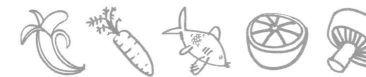

AFTER-SCHOOL SNACKS AND LUNCHBOX TREATS

Chicken, tuna, or cheese sandwich on whole-grain bread

Banana or honey sandwich on whole-grain bread

Whole-grain toast with peanut butter

Crackers, oat cakes, or rice cakes with a little cheese

Yogurt drink

Slice or cubes of cheese

Nuts (e.g., peanuts, cashews, almonds)

Sesame snaps

Crudités (e.g., carrots, red and green peppers, cucumbers, celery)

Hummus (see recipe on page 193)

Fresh fruit (e.g., apple slices, pear, oranges, grapes, strawberries)

Carton of yogurt and fresh fruit

Dried fruit (e.g., raisins, apricots, apple rings, mango) and cheese

Mini pancake or scone

Whole-grain breakfast cereal with milk

Plain popcorn

Apple Muffins (see recipe on page 194)

Fruit Muffins (see recipe on page 194)

Banana Muffins (see recipe on page 195)

Apple Spice Cake (see recipe on page 196)

Carrot Cake (see recipe on page 197)

Fruit Cake (see recipe on page 198)

Ginger Spice Cake (see recipe on page 199)

Whole-Wheat Raisin Cookies (see recipe on page 200)

Apricot Bars (see recipe on page 200)

Smoothie (e.g., Banana Smoothie; see recipe on page 203)

Milkshake (e.g., Strawberry and Banana Milkshake; see recipe on page 206)

Accompany all snacks with a glass of water or diluted fruit juice.

AFTER-SPORT SNACKS

Bananas

Fresh fruit (e.g., grapes, apples, oranges, pears)

Dried fruit (e.g., raisins, apricots, dates)

Fruit bars

Crackers and rice cakes with bananas or cheese

Roll, sandwich bread, English muffin, or bagel with
honey or jam

Cereal bar or granola bar (e.g., Cereal Bar; see recipe on page 201)

Energy bar

Fruit yogurt

Milkshake (see recipes on pages 202–206)

Smoothie (see recipes on pages 202–206)

Banana Muffins (see recipe on page 195)

Banana Loaf (see recipe on page 195)

Whole-Wheat Raisin Cookies (see recipe on page 200)

Accompany all snacks with a glass of water, diluted fruit juice, or isotonic sports drink.

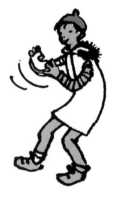

CHAPTER 14

🌶🥒🥕🥔🍅🍄🍓

Main Meals

Chicken Baked in Tomato Sauce

Anything in tomato sauce will be a hit with most children, so you can use this dish as a good opportunity to disguise extra vegetables.

To balance the meal, serve with baked potatoes and carrots.

4 chicken legs and thighs (about 1 pound)

2 tablespoons olive oil, divided

1 small onion, chopped

2 garlic cloves, minced

¼ cup each chopped red and green bell pepper

1 can (14 ounces) chopped tomatoes, undrained

1 tablespoon each chopped fresh basil, parsley, and chives, or 1 tablespoon of dried herbs

Salt and freshly ground black pepper, to taste

Preheat the oven to 350°F.

Cook chicken pieces in 1 tablespoon oil in medium skillet over medium heat until browned, about 5 minutes. Remove with a slotted spoon and place in a small casserole or baking dish.

Add remaining 1 tablespoon oil to the skillet and sauté the onion and garlic for 3 minutes. Add bell peppers and sauté 2 minutes longer. Add tomatoes and liquid and herbs and heat to boiling; reduce heat and simmer, uncovered, 5 minutes. Season to taste with salt and pepper.

Spoon tomato sauce over the chicken and bake, covered, until chicken is cooked and tender, about 45 minutes.

Makes 4 servings.

Per serving: 536.0 calories / 48.5 g protein / 7.7 g carbohydrate / 1.8 g fiber / 33.6 g total fat / 9.2 g saturated fat / 216.3 mg cholesterol / 373.1 mg sodium

NUTRITIONAL ANALYSIS PER SERVING

Vitamin A	159.3 RE	Vitamin D	0.0 µg	Thiamin (B-1)	0.1 mg	Vitamin E	1.8 mg
Riboflavin (B-2)	0.4 mg	Calcium	46.9 mg	Niacin	11.5 mg	Iron	3.0 mg
Vitamin B-6	0.7 mg	Phosphorus	323.5 mg	Vitamin B-12	0.5 µg	Magnesium	46.9 mg
Folate (total)	26.2 µg	Zinc	4.6 mg	Vitamin C	42.7 mg	Potassium	501.0 mg

Chicken Curry

Make this dish more nutritious by adding extra vegetables to the curry sauce. Adjust the amount of curry powder according to your children's taste.

1 pound boneless, skinless chicken breast halves, cut into ½-inch strips

1 tablespoon olive oil

1 small onion, chopped

1 clove garlic, minced

1–2 teaspoons curry powder (or paste)

1 can (14 ounces) chopped tomatoes, undrained

1 cup small cauliflower florets

1 cup sliced carrots

1 cup frozen peas

Salt and freshly ground black pepper, to taste

¼ cup golden raisins

Cook chicken in olive oil in large skillet over medium heat until browned, about 5 minutes; remove from skillet and reserve. Add onion and garlic to the skillet and sauté until tender, about 5 minutes. Stir in curry powder, tomatoes and liquid, and vegetables. Heat to boiling; reduce heat and simmer, covered, 10 minutes. Season to taste with salt and pepper.

Add reserved chicken and the raisins to the skillet and simmer, uncovered, until hot through, 5 to 10 minutes.

Makes 4 servings.

To balance the meal, serve with basmati rice and warmed pita bread.

PER SERVING: 267.4 calories / 31.1 g protein / 24.5 g carbohydrate / 5.5 g fiber / 5.4 g total fat / 0.9 g saturated fat / 65.7 mg cholesterol / 324.5 mg sodium

NUTRITIONAL ANALYSIS PER SERVING

Vitamin A	908.9 RE	Vitamin D	0.0 µg	Thiamin (B-1)	0.2 mg	Vitamin E	0.9 mg
Riboflavin (B-2)	0.2 mg	Calcium	60.5 mg	Niacin	11.2 mg	Iron	2.4 mg
Vitamin B-6	0.7 mg	Phosphorus	241.4 mg	Vitamin B-12	0.3 µg	Magnesium	44.1 mg
Folate (total)	38.4 µg	Zinc	1.4 mg	Vitamin C	29.9 mg	Potassium	499.7 mg

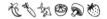

Pasta Turkey Bolognese

Ground turkey is used in place of beef. It is high in protein and low in fat. Bolognese sauce is a good way of hiding vegetables and beans.

12 ounces ground turkey

1 tablespoon olive oil

½ cup chopped onion

2 ribs celery, chopped

2 carrots, grated

1 can (14 ounces) chopped tomatoes, undrained

1 can (15 ounces) red kidney beans, rinsed, drained

1 teaspoon dried Italian seasoning

Salt and freshly ground black pepper, to taste

6–8 ounces spaghetti or other pasta, cooked, warm (adjust the quantity according to the child's appetite)

Cook turkey in oil in large skillet over medium heat until browned, about 5 minutes. Add onion, celery, and carrots and sauté until tender, 5 to 7 minutes.

Stir in tomatoes and liquid, beans, and Italian seasoning; heat to boiling. Reduce heat and simmer, uncovered, 5 minutes; season to taste with salt and pepper. Serve over spaghetti.

Makes 4 servings.

To balance the meal, serve with steamed broccoli or spring cabbage.

PER SERVING: 448.4 calories / 27.9 g protein / 57.3 g carbohydrate / 10.3 g fiber / 12.0 g total fat / 2.6 g saturated fat / 67.3 mg cholesterol / 670.0 mg sodium

NUTRITIONAL ANALYSIS PER SERVING

Vitamin A	876.8	RE	Vitamin D	0.0	µg	Thiamin (B-1)	0.5	mg	Vitamin E	1.1	mg
Riboflavin (B-2)	0.4	mg	Calcium	78.4	mg	Niacin	5.6	mg	Iron	4.2	mg
Vitamin B-6	0.4	mg	Phosphorus	281.2	mg	Vitamin B-12	0.2	µg	Magnesium	67.9	mg
Folate (total)	157.3	µg	Zinc	2.9	mg	Vitamin C	16.6	mg	Potassium	630.9	mg

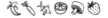

Golden Baked Chicken

This is one of the easiest and healthiest ways to cook chicken—children will love it!

½ cup all-purpose flour

1 tablespoon paprika

4 boneless, skinless chicken breasts halves (about 4 ounces each)

2 tablespoons olive oil

Salt and freshly ground black pepper, to taste

Preheat the oven to 350°F.

Place flour and paprika in a plastic bag. Add the chicken breasts and shake until the chicken is well coated.

Pour olive oil into a baking dish. Add the chicken breasts and turn carefully to coat lightly with oil; sprinkle lightly with salt and pepper. Cover with foil and bake until cooked and tender, about 20 minutes.

To balance the meal, serve with green beans and mashed potatoes.

Remove the foil and bake 10 minutes longer, until the chicken is golden brown.

Makes 4 servings.

PER SERVING: 245.2 calories / 28.0 g protein / 12.8 g carbohydrate / 1.0 g fiber / 8.4 g total fat / 1.3 g saturated fat / 65.7 mg cholesterol / 60.0 mg sodium

NUTRITIONAL ANALYSIS PER SERVING

Vitamin A	100.5	RE	Vitamin D	0.0	µg	Thiamin (B-1)	0.2	mg	Vitamin E	1.0	mg
Riboflavin (B-2)	0.2	mg	Calcium	17.0	mg	Niacin	11.3	mg	Iron	1.9	mg
Vitamin B-6	0.6	mg	Phosphorus	200.1	mg	Vitamin B-12	0.3	µg	Magnesium	30.1	mg
Folate (total)	33.0	µg	Zinc	1.1	mg	Vitamin C	2.2	mg	Potassium	285.0	mg

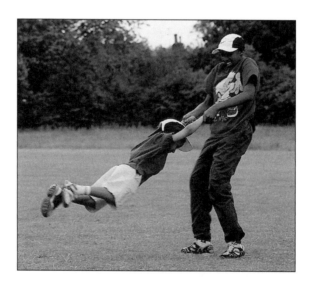

Chicken and Vegetable Packets

These pies are made with fillo pastry (also spelled phyllo, and available in the supermarket's freezer section), which contains less fat than traditional piecrust pastry. You can substitute different vegetables for those suggested in the recipe; they will count towards the 5 daily servings of vegetables and fruit recommended for children.

To balance the meal, serve with Oven Potato Wedges (page 182) and a green vegetable.

12 ounces skinless, boneless chicken breast, cut into scant ½-inch pieces

1 tablespoon olive oil

1 cup sliced small button mushrooms

¾ cup finely chopped zucchini

¾ cup thinly sliced carrots

1 tablespoon cornstarch

1 cup milk

Salt and freshly ground black pepper, to taste

12 sheets fillo pastry

Olive oil or vegetable cooking spray

Preheat the oven to 375°F.

Sauté chicken in oil in large skillet 3 minutes. Add the vegetables and sauté until tender, about 5 minutes. Stir in cornstarch. Slowly stir in milk; heat to boiling, stirring continuously, until the sauce has thickened, about 1 minute. Remove from heat; season to taste with salt and pepper.

Spray 1 sheet fillo lightly with olive oil spray and top with second sheet of fillo; spray lightly and top with third sheet of fillo. Spoon ¼ the chicken mixture along center of fillo; fold into a packet, tucking ends in. Repeat with remaining fillo and chicken mixture to make 4 packets. Spray tops of packets with olive oil spray and place on baking sheet. Bake, uncovered, 15–20 minutes, until golden brown.

Makes 4 servings.

PER SERVING: 348.0 calories / 26.7 g protein / 38.1 g carbohydrate / 2.2 g fiber / 9.2 g total fat / 2.3 g saturated fat / 54.2 mg cholesterol / 363.3 mg sodium

NUTRITIONAL ANALYSIS PER SERVING

Vitamin A	674.4 RE	Vitamin D	0.9 µg	Thiamin (B-1)	0.4 mg	Vitamin E	1.3 mg
Riboflavin (B-2)	0.5 mg	Calcium	97.8 mg	Niacin	11.0 mg	Iron	2.7 mg
Vitamin B-6	0.5 mg	Phosphorus	264.6 mg	Vitamin B-12	0.5 µg	Magnesium	41.1 mg
Folate (total)	68.5 µg	Zinc	1.4 mg	Vitamin C	6.3 mg	Potassium	490.6 mg

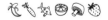

Toad-and-Vegetables-in-the-Hole

This variation on a British dish called Toad-in-the-Hole includes tasty root vegetables, which add extra vitamins and fiber to the meal. It is also a good dish to serve to vegetarians, as vegetarian sausages can be used.

4 medium carrots

1 medium parsnip

8 ounces butternut squash

2 tablespoons canola oil

4 lean beef, turkey, or
vegetarian sausages

1 cup all-purpose flour

1 egg

1 cup milk

Preheat the oven to 375°F.

Peel vegetables and cut into 1-inch chunks. Place in a roasting pan, drizzle with the oil, and toss to coat. Bake, uncovered, 20 minutes.

Pierce the sausages with a fork; add to the roasting pan and bake another 10 minutes. Transfer vegetables and sausages to a baking pan.

Process the flour, egg, and milk in a blender until smooth. Pour the batter over the vegetables and sausages and bake 40 minutes, or until the batter has risen and is crisp on the outside.

Makes 4 servings.

To balance the meal, add a green vegetable.

PER SERVING: 451.7 calories / 25.0 g protein / 46.1 g carbohydrate / 5.1 g fiber / 19.7 g total fat / 4.2 g saturated fat / 112.0 mg cholesterol / 928.4 mg sodium

NUTRITIONAL ANALYSIS PER SERVING

Vitamin A	2,115.8 RE	Vitamin D	0.8 µg	Thiamin (B-1)	0.4 mg	Vitamin E	1.9 mg
Riboflavin (B-2)	0.4 mg	Calcium	157.3 mg	Niacin	3.3 mg	Iron	3.8 mg
Vitamin B-6	0.2 mg	Phosphorus	175.5 mg	Vitamin B-12	0.4 µg	Magnesium	48.2 mg
Folate (total)	107.5 µg	Zinc	1.0 mg	Vitamin C	17.0 mg	Potassium	628.6 mg

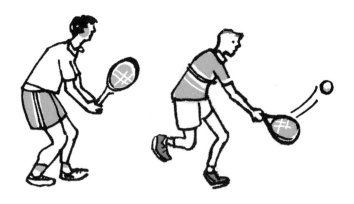

Pasta with Corn and Tuna

This dish is quick to prepare and makes a good midweek standby. It's also good eaten cold as a lunchbox salad.

8 ounces pasta, any shape (adjust the quantity according to the child's appetite)

1 small onion, chopped

1 garlic clove, minced

1 tablespoon olive oil

1 can (14 ounces) chopped tomatoes, undrained

1 tablespoon tomato paste

½ cup whole kernel corn

1 can (7 ounces) tuna packed in water, drained and flaked

1 teaspoon dried basil leaves

Salt and freshly ground black pepper, to taste

Cook the pasta in boiling water according to the package directions. Drain.

Meanwhile, sauté onion and garlic in oil in a large skillet for 4–5 minutes or until onion is soft. Stir in the tomatoes and liquid, tomato paste, and corn, and cook, uncovered, over medium heat for 5 minutes. Add the tuna and basil and heat through; season to taste with salt and pepper. Serve over pasta.

Makes 4 servings.

To balance the meal, serve with broccoli or brussels sprouts.

PER SERVING: 350.7 calories / 22.4 g protein / 53.7 g carbohydrate / 3.6 g fiber / 5.2 g total fat / 0.7 g saturated fat / 14.9 mg cholesterol / 411.7 mg sodium

NUTRITIONAL ANALYSIS PER SERVING

Vitamin A	41.2	RE	Vitamin D	0.0	µg	Thiamin (B-1)	0.4	mg	Vitamin E	1.1	mg
Riboflavin (B-2)	0.3	mg	Calcium	40.9	mg	Niacin	9.8	mg	Iron	3.3	mg
Vitamin B-6	0.3	mg	Phosphorus	183.0	mg	Vitamin B-12	1.5	µg	Magnesium	48.4	mg
Folate (total)	126.2	µg	Zinc	1.3	mg	Vitamin C	15.6	mg	Potassium	289.1	mg

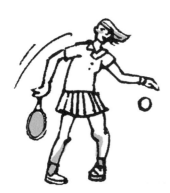

Pasta with Ham and Mushroom Sauce

8 ounces pasta shells (adjust the quantity according to the child's appetite)

1 tablespoon olive oil

4 ounces reduced-sodium ham, chopped

4 ounces small fresh mushrooms, halved

1 tablespoons cornstarch

1 cup milk

1 teaspoon dried oregano

Salt and freshly ground black pepper, to taste

Cook the pasta in boiling water according to the package directions. Drain.

Meanwhile, heat the olive oil in a large skillet. Cook the ham and mushrooms over medium heat for 4–5 minutes. Stir in the cornstarch mixed with a little milk; blend until smooth. Gradually add the rest of the milk, stirring continuously; heat to boiling, stirring until thickened. Stir in oregano; season to taste with salt and pepper. Combine with the pasta and serve.

Makes 4 servings.

To balance the meal, serve with carrots and a green vegetable.

PER SERVING: 317.2 calories / 14.7 g protein / 49.1 g carbohydrate / 1.9 g fiber / 6.7 g total fat / 1.8 g saturated fat / 18.4 mg cholesterol / 262.5 mg sodium

NUTRITIONAL ANALYSIS PER SERVING

Vitamin A	25.6 RE	Vitamin D	1.1 µg	Thiamin (B-1)	0.4 mg	Vitamin E	0.6 mg
Riboflavin (B-2)	0.4 mg	Calcium	87.9 mg	Niacin	3.9 mg	Iron	2.3 mg
Vitamin B-6	0.1 mg	Phosphorus	154.7 mg	Vitamin B-12	0.3 µg	Magnesium	33.5 mg
Folate (total)	119.0 µg	Zinc	1.1 mg	Vitamin C	1.0 mg	Potassium	214.4 mg

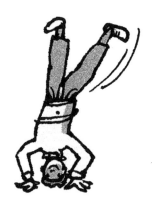

Pasta and Tuna Bake

This recipe makes a balanced meal in itself. The tuna and milk provide protein, the pasta provides energy-giving carbohydrate, and the vegetables provide vitamins and fiber.

To balance the meal, serve fresh fruit for dessert.

8 ounces pasta shells (adjust the quantity according to the child's appetite)

1 tablespoon olive oil

1 small onion, sliced

2 ribs celery, chopped

1 small green bell pepper, chopped

4 ounces frozen peas

1 tablespoon butter

1 tablespoon cornstarch

1 cup milk

1 can (7 ounces) tuna in water, drained

1 tablespoon chopped parsley

Preheat the oven to 375°F.

Cook the pasta in boiling water according to the package directions. Drain.

In a nonstick skillet, heat the olive oil. Sauté the onion for 3 minutes on medium heat until translucent; add the celery, bell pepper, and peas and sauté 5 minutes longer.

Melt butter in a medium saucepan, stir in cornstarch, then stir in milk slowly. Heat over a high heat to boiling, stirring constantly; boil, stirring until thickened, about 1 minute.

Spread half the vegetables onto the bottom of a 9 x 9–inch baking dish. Cover with half the pasta, tuna, and white sauce, sprinkling parsley between each layer. Repeat with remaining ingredients, finishing with white sauce on top. Bake, uncovered, until hot through, about 20 minutes.

Makes 4 servings.

PER SERVING: 404.1 calories / 24.1 g protein / 55.9 g carbohydrate / 4.2 g fiber / 9.0 g total fat / 3.3 g saturated fat / 27.4 mg cholesterol / 254.1 mg sodium

NUTRITIONAL ANALYSIS PER SERVING

Vitamin A	94.6 RE	Vitamin D	0.7 µg	Thiamin (B-1)	0.5 mg	Vitamin E	1.3 mg
Riboflavin (B-2)	0.4 mg	Calcium	112.6 mg	Niacin	10.1 mg	Iron	3.1 mg
Vitamin B-6	0.4 mg	Phosphorus	252.2 mg	Vitamin B-12	1.8 µg	Magnesium	58.0 mg
Folate (total)	149.3 µg	Zinc	1.6 mg	Vitamin C	30.5 mg	Potassium	417.7 mg

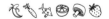

Lasagne

Choosing lean ground beef keeps the saturated-fat content of this recipe to a minimum. In-clude other varieties of vegetables, such as mushrooms and spinach, instead of the celery and pepper, if you wish. This dish is a good way of hiding those vegetables!

1 small onion, chopped

1 rib celery, chopped

1 small red bell pepper, chopped

1 tablespoon olive oil

8 ounces lean ground beef or ground turkey

1 can (14 ounces) chopped tomatoes, undrained

2 tablespoons tomato paste

1 teaspoon dried basil or oregano

Salt and freshly ground black pepper, to taste

8 no-boil lasagne noodles

3 ounces shredded mozzarella cheese

Preheat the oven to 350°F.

Sauté the onion, celery, and bell pepper in oil in large skillet 3 to 4 minutes. Add beef and cook over medium heat, stirring frequently, 5–6 minutes, until the meat is browned. Drain off any fat. Add the tomatoes and liq-uid, tomato paste, and oregano. Season with salt and pepper to taste.

Place 4 lasagne noodles in the bottom of an oiled 13 x 9–inch baking dish. Spoon one-third of the meat mixture on top. Repeat the layers, finishing with a layer of the meat mixture. Sprinkle with mozzarella. Bake, uncov-ered, 30 minutes, until the lasagne is hot through.

Makes 4 servings.

To balance the meal, add fresh fruit for dessert.

PER SERVING: 396.5 calories / 23.7 g protein / 37.4 g carbohydrate / 4.0 g fiber / 17.3 g total fat / 6.6 g saturated fat / 49.6 mg cholesterol / 464.4 mg sodium

NUTRITIONAL ANALYSIS PER SERVING

Vitamin A	277.4 RE	Vitamin D	0.0 µg	Thiamin (B-1)	0.1 mg	Vitamin E	1.3 mg
Riboflavin (B-2)	0.2 mg	Calcium	187.1 mg	Niacin	2.9 mg	Iron	2.1 mg
Vitamin B-6	0.2 mg	Phosphorus	106.0 mg	Vitamin B-12	0.9 µg	Magnesium	23.7 mg
Folate (total)	19.3 µg	Zinc	2.6 mg	Vitamin C	72.3 mg	Potassium	384.6 mg

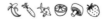

Chili con Carne

This version of the classic dish smuggles in extra vegetables. You may use any type of lean ground meat, such as turkey, beef, or pork.

8 ounces lean ground turkey, beef, or pork

1 small onion, chopped

1 garlic clove, minced

1 small green bell pepper, chopped

1 rib celery, chopped

3 ounces button mushrooms, whole or cut in half

1 teaspoon paprika

1 pinch chili powder (adjust according to the child's tastes)

½ teaspoon ground cumin

1 can (14 ounces) diced tomatoes, undrained

2 tablespoons tomato paste

1½ cups beef broth or water

1 can (15 ounces) red kidney beans, rinsed, drained

Salt and freshly ground pepper, to taste

Cook the meat in a greased skillet over medium heat until browned, about 5 minutes. Drain off any fat.

Add the onion, garlic, bell pepper, celery, and mushrooms and sauté until tender, about 5 minutes. Add the spices and cook 1 minute longer. Add the tomatoes and liquid, tomato paste, broth, and beans. Cover and heat to boiling; reduce heat and simmer, covered, for a minimum of 20 to 30 minutes; season to taste with salt and pepper.

Makes 4 servings.

To balance the meal, serve with boiled rice and a green vegetable.

PER SERVING: 214.9 calories / 21.5 g protein / 28.8 g carbohydrate / 9.6 g fiber / 1.6 g total fat / 0.4 g saturated fat / 22.5 mg cholesterol / 976.0 mg sodium

NUTRITIONAL ANALYSIS PER SERVING

Vitamin A	107.6 RE	Vitamin D	0.4 µg	Thiamin (B-1)	0.2 mg	Vitamin E	0.8 mg
Riboflavin (B-2)	0.2 mg	Calcium	95.9 mg	Niacin	1.8 mg	Iron	3.3 mg
Vitamin B-6	0.2 mg	Phosphorus	143.8 mg	Vitamin B-12	0.0 µg	Magnesium	43.2 mg
Folate (total)	71.4 µg	Zinc	0.9 mg	Vitamin C	42.3 mg	Potassium	563.1 mg

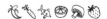

Chicken and Mixed Pepper Risotto

Peppers are bursting with vitamin C and other antioxidants. This recipe is a great way of introducing them to children.

1 tablespoon olive oil

1 small onion, chopped

1 small red bell pepper, cut into thin strips

1 small yellow bell pepper, cut into thin strips

6 ounces Arborio or long-grain rice

3 cups chicken or vegetable stock

4 ounces cooked chicken, chopped

1 ounce Parmesan cheese, grated

Handful of fresh chives or parsley, if available

Heat the olive oil in a large saucepan. Sauté the onion and peppers until tender, about 7 minutes. Add the rice and cook for 2–3 minutes until the rice is translucent. Add the stock and heat to boiling. Reduce heat and simmer, partially covered, 20 to 25 minutes until the rice is tender and the liquid has been absorbed, stirring frequently. Add a little more stock if the risotto becomes dry.

Add the chicken and half the Parmesan; cook 3 to 4 minutes. Serve topped with the remaining Parmesan and herbs.

Makes 4 servings.

To balance the meal, add fresh fruit for dessert.

PER SERVING: 301.2 calories / 15.5 g protein / 44.8 g carbohydrate / 2.2 g fiber / 6.8 g total fat / 2.0 g saturated fat / 28.0 mg cholesterol / 473.7 mg sodium

NUTRITIONAL ANALYSIS PER SERVING

Vitamin A	284.7 RE	Vitamin D	0.1 µg	Thiamin (B-1)	0.1 mg	Vitamin E	0.8 mg
Riboflavin (B-2)	0.1 mg	Calcium	110.6 mg	Niacin	3.1 mg	Iron	1.3 mg
Vitamin B-6	0.3 mg	Phosphorus	308.5 mg	Vitamin B-12	0.2 µg	Magnesium	21.4 mg
Folate (total)	24.2 µg	Zinc	0.7 mg	Vitamin C	143.6 mg	Potassium	447.4 mg

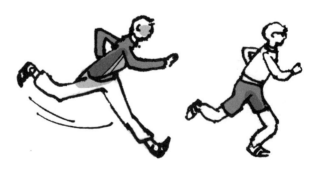

Fish Cakes

All fish is rich in protein and important minerals. Salmon, in particular, is rich in the essential omega-3 fatty acids, important for brain development and physical activity.

1 pound potatoes, peeled

1 pound salmon or cod fillets, skinned

4 tablespoons butter

¼ cup milk

1 tablespoon chopped parsley

Salt and freshly ground black pepper, to taste

1 to 2 tablespoons olive oil

Cut the potatoes into quarters and boil, covered, in water in large saucepan until tender, about 15 minutes; drain.

Meanwhile, poach the fish, covered, in water in large skillet for 10 minutes. Drain and flake the fish, carefully removing all the bones.

Mash the potatoes with the butter, milk, and parsley; season to taste with salt and pepper. Mix in the flaked fish. Shape into 4 or 8 cakes. Cook in oil in large skillet over medium heat until browned, about 4 minutes on each side. Drain on paper towels.

Makes 4 large or 8 small fish cakes (4 servings).

To balance the meal, serve with carrots and peas.

PER SERVING: 425.4 calories / 25.1 g protein / 18.6 g carbohydrate / 2.8 g fiber / 27.5 g total fat / 10.4 g saturated fat / 98.1 mg cholesterol / 162.4 mg sodium

NUTRITIONAL ANALYSIS PER SERVING

Vitamin A	97.0 RE	Vitamin D	0.4 µg	Thiamin (B-1)	0.5 mg	Vitamin E	0.7 mg
Riboflavin (B-2)	0.2 mg	Calcium	46.4 mg	Niacin	9.8 mg	Iron	1.1 mg
Vitamin B-6	0.9 mg	Phosphorus	352.8 mg	Vitamin B-12	2.6 µg	Magnesium	58.0 mg
Folate (total)	51.1 µg	Zinc	0.9 mg	Vitamin C	27.4 mg	Potassium	903.6 mg

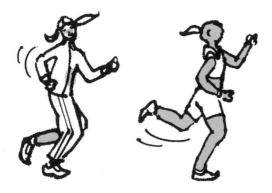

Bean and Tuna Salad

The beans provide protein, B vitamins, iron, and fiber.

1 can (15 ounces) cannellini or butter beans, rinsed, drained

2 small tomatoes, cubed

1 can (3½ ounces) tuna in water, drained and flaked

4 ounces green beans, cooked and cooled

1 tablespoon red wine vinegar

2 tablespoons olive oil

Handful of chopped fresh chives or parsley

Mix the canned beans, tomatoes, tuna, and green beans in a bowl; add combined vinegar, oil, and herbs and toss. Makes 4 servings.

To balance the meal, add cooked pasta.

PER SERVING: 202.1 calories / 12.8 g protein / 20.9 g carbohydrate / 6.8 g fiber / 7.8 g total fat / 1.1 g saturated fat / 7.4 mg cholesterol / 310.7 mg sodium

NUTRITIONAL ANALYSIS PER SERVING

Vitamin A	233.4 RE	Vitamin D	0.0 µg	Thiamin (B-1)	0.1 mg	Vitamin E	1.4 mg
Riboflavin (B-2)	0.1 mg	Calcium	88.4 mg	Niacin	4.1 mg	Iron	3.0 mg
Vitamin B-6	0.2 mg	Phosphorus	88.1 mg	Vitamin B-12	0.7 µg	Magnesium	37.0 mg
Folate (total)	59.0 µg	Zinc	0.6 mg	Vitamin C	34.5 mg	Potassium	376.2 mg

CHAPTER 15

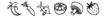

Meatless Main Meals

Vegetarian Spaghetti Bolognese

Lentils are substituted for the meat in the Bolognese sauce. They provide plenty of protein, iron, fiber, and B vitamins and make a super-tasty main course.

1 tablespoon olive oil

1 small onion, chopped

2 medium carrots, shredded

1 large zucchini, finely chopped

1 can (14 ounces) chopped tomatoes, undrained

1 can (15 ounces) lentils or 4 ounces dried lentils, soaked and cooked

1 teaspoon mixed dried herbs

8 ounces spaghetti (adjust the quantity according to the child's appetite)

2 tablespoons olive oil, divided

2 tablespoons grated Parmesan cheese

Heat the olive oil in a large skillet. Add the onion, carrots, and zucchini and sauté until tender, about 5 minutes. Add the tomatoes and liquid, lentils, and herbs and heat to boiling; reduce heat and simmer, uncovered, until the sauce thickens slightly, about 5 minutes.

Meanwhile, cook the spaghetti in boiling water according to the package directions. Drain and toss in olive oil. Serve sauce over the spaghetti and sprinkle with the Parmesan cheese.

Makes 4 servings.

To balance the meal, serve fresh fruit for dessert.

PER SERVING: 443.7 calories / 17.3 g protein / 67.1 g carbohydrate / 11.5 g fiber / 12.3 g total fat / 2.0 g saturated fat / 2.2 mg cholesterol / 523.2 mg sodium

NUTRITIONAL ANALYSIS PER SERVING

Vitamin A	893.9 RE	Vitamin D	0.0 µg	Thiamin (B-1)	0.4 mg	Vitamin E	1.6 mg
Riboflavin (B-2)	0.3 mg	Calcium	86.1 mg	Niacin	3.3 mg	Iron	4.7 mg
Vitamin B-6	0.2 mg	Phosphorus	127.2 mg	Vitamin B-12	0.1 µg	Magnesium	38.8 mg
Folate (total)	135.8 µg	Zinc	1.0 mg	Vitamin C	25.6 mg	Potassium	296.4 mg

Pasta Shells with Tomato and Peppers

This is one of the quickest standby dishes in my house! You can add other vegetables, such as mushrooms, zucchini, or green beans, to the tomato sauce instead of peppers.

1 tablespoon olive oil

1 small onion, chopped

2 garlic cloves, minced

1 small red or green bell pepper, chopped

1 can (14 ounces) chopped tomatoes, undrained

2 tablespoons tomato paste

1 teaspoon dried basil

Salt and freshly ground black pepper, to taste

Pinch of sugar

8 ounces pasta shells (adjust the quantity according to the child's appetite)

3 ounces Cheddar cheese, grated

Heat the olive oil in a large skillet. Add the onion, garlic, and bell pepper and sauté for 5 minutes, or until the vegetables have softened.

Add the tomatoes and liquid, tomato paste, and basil and heat to boiling. Reduce heat and simmer, uncovered, until slightly thickened, about 5 minutes. Season to taste with salt and pepper, and sugar.

Meanwhile, cook the pasta shells in boiling water according to the package directions. Drain. Combine the sauce with the pasta and sprinkle with the cheese.

Makes 4 servings.

To balance the meal, serve with broccoli or brussels sprouts.

PER SERVING: 374.1 calories / 14.8 g protein / 52.5 g carbohydrate / 3.5 g fiber / 12.0 g total fat / 5.0 g saturated fat / 22.3 mg cholesterol / 407 mg sodium

NUTRITIONAL ANALYSIS PER SERVING

Vitamin A	266.9 RE	Vitamin D	0.1 µg	Thiamin (B-1)	0.6 mg	Vitamin E	1.1 mg
Riboflavin (B-2)	0.4 mg	Calcium	183.3 mg	Niacin	3.6 mg	Iron	3.0 mg
Vitamin B-6	0.2 mg	Phosphorus	134.8 mg	Vitamin B-12	0.2 µg	Magnesium	17.6 mg
Folate (total)	136.4 µg	Zinc	0.9 mg	Vitamin C	72.5 mg	Potassium	224.4 mg

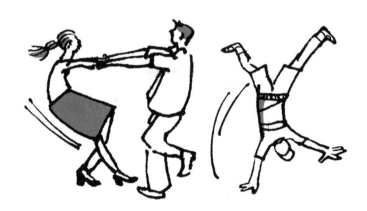

Marvelous Macaroni and Cheese

Macaroni and cheese is popular with most children. Here's a more nutritious version with peas and mushrooms; but it also works well with broad beans, carrots, and red kidney beans

To balance the meal, serve with green beans.

8 ounces elbow macaroni (adjust the quantity according to the child's appetite)

2 ounces frozen peas

2 tablespoons butter

2 ounces button mushrooms, sliced

3 tablespoons cornstarch

1 cup milk (skim or part skim is preferable to whole)

½ teaspoon Dijon mustard

3 ounces aged Cheddar cheese, shredded

Salt and freshly ground black pepper, to taste

Preheat the oven to 400°F.

Cook the macaroni in boiling water according to the package directions, adding the frozen peas during the last 3 minutes of cooking time. Drain.

Heat the butter in a large saucepan. Add the mushrooms and sauté for 2 minutes. Blend the cornstarch with a little of the milk in a bowl until smooth; gradually add the remainder of the milk. Add the milk to the mushrooms in the pan and heat to boiling, stirring continuously until thickened, about 1 minute.

Remove from heat. Stir in mustard and half the cheese; season to taste with salt and pepper. Stir in the macaroni and peas. Spoon mixture into a baking dish and sprinkle with remaining cheese. Bake, uncovered, for 15–20 minutes until the top is bubbling and golden.

Makes 4 servings.

PER SERVING: 407.7 calories / 15.8 g protein / 53.9 g carbohydrate / 3.0 g fiber / 14.0 g total fat / 8.2 g saturated fat / 38.8 mg cholesterol / 225.0 mg sodium

NUTRITIONAL ANALYSIS PER SERVING

Vitamin A	141.6 RE	Vitamin D	1.0 µg	Thiamin (B-1)	0.5 mg	Vitamin E	0.3 mg
Riboflavin (B-2)	0.4 mg	Calcium	236.4 mg	Niacin	3.9 mg	Iron	2.3 mg
Vitamin B-6	0.1 mg	Phosphorus	196.2 mg	Vitamin B-12	0.5 µg	Magnesium	17.4 mg
Folate (total)	139.2 µg	Zinc	1.1 mg	Vitamin C	1.7 mg	Potassium	178.4 mg

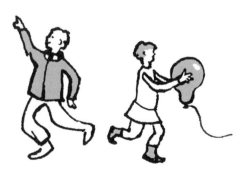

Penne with Cheese and Broccoli

Broccoli is full of vitamin C, folate, and other powerful antioxidants. This recipe is a tasty way of getting your children to eat it!

8 ounces penne pasta (adjust the quantity according to the child's appetite)

8 ounces broccoli florets

1 tablespoon olive oil

1 small onion, sliced

1 tablespoon cornstarch

1 cup milk

2 ounces aged Cheddar cheese, shredded

Cook the pasta in boiling water according to the package directions, adding the broccoli during the last 3 minutes of cooking time. Drain.

In a large saucepan, sauté the onion in the olive oil for 5 minutes until softened. Blend the cornstarch with a little of the milk in a bowl until smooth. Gradually add the remainder of the milk. Slowly add to the saucepan and heat to boiling, stirring continuously until the sauce has thickened, about 1 minute; stir in the cheese. Combine with the pasta and broccoli.

To balance the meal, serve with carrots or sliced tomatoes.

Makes 4 servings.

PER SERVING: 364.3 calories / 14.4 g protein / 52.8 g carbohydrate / 3.1 g fiber / 10.2 g total fat / 4.3 g saturated fat / 19.8 mg cholesterol / 130.0 mg sodium

NUTRITIONAL ANALYSIS PER SERVING

Vitamin A	97.0 RE	Vitamin D	0.7 µg	Thiamin (B-1)	0.4 mg	Vitamin E	0.7 mg
Riboflavin (B-2)	0.4 mg	Calcium	203.2 mg	Niacin	2.6 mg	Iron	2.1 mg
Vitamin B-6	0.1 mg	Phosphorus	209.9 mg	Vitamin B-12	0.4 µg	Magnesium	36.6 mg
Folate (total)	89.6 µg	Zinc	1.4 mg	Vitamin C	22.6 mg	Potassium	172.6 mg

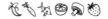

Chickpea and Spinach Pasta

This is a great way of including spinach in your children's diet. It is rich in iron, folate, and vitamin C.

1 can (14 ounces) chickpeas, rinsed and drained

1 cup spaghetti sauce

¼ cup water

8 ounces penne pasta

4 ounces baby spinach leaves

Salt and freshly ground black pepper, to taste

1 ounce Parmesan cheese, grated

Heat chickpeas, spaghetti sauce, and water to boiling in a medium saucepan; remove from heat and cover.

Meanwhile, cook the pasta in boiling water according to the package directions. Drain. Stir in the spinach and allow it to wilt. Spoon the pasta into a serving dish; stir in the chickpea mixture. Season to taste with salt and pepper. Top with grated Parmesan.

Makes 4 servings.

To balance the meal, serve fresh fruit for dessert.

PER SERVING: 386.1 calories / 16.4 g protein / 70.4 g carbohydrate / 7.2 g fiber / 4.4 g total fat / 1.5 g saturated fat / 6.2 mg cholesterol / 744.2 mg sodium

NUTRITIONAL ANALYSIS PER SERVING

Vitamin A	169.0 RE	Vitamin D	0.1 µg	Thiamin (B-1)	0.4 mg	Vitamin E	0.1 mg
Riboflavin (B-2)	0.3 mg	Calcium	150.1 mg	Niacin	2.9 mg	Iron	5.5 mg
Vitamin B-6	0.6 mg	Phosphorus	226.5 mg	Vitamin B-12	0.2 µg	Magnesium	77.2 mg
Folate (total)	146.0 µg	Zinc	2.2 mg	Vitamin C	11.5 mg	Potassium	325.9 mg

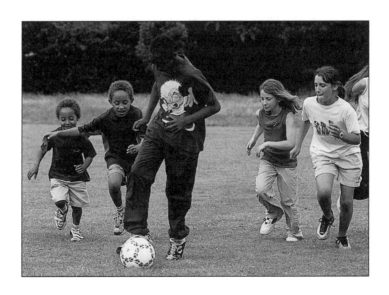

Red Kidney Bean Lasagne

This dish is a firm favorite with my children. The combination of pasta, vegetables, red kidney beans, and cheese makes it a near-perfect balanced meal.

1 tablespoon olive oil

1 small onion, chopped

1 small red bell pepper, chopped

2 ounces mushrooms, chopped

1 small zucchini, sliced

1 teaspoon dried basil

1 can (14 ounces) red kidney beans, rinsed and drained

1 can (14 ounces) crushed tomatoes, undrained

Salt and freshly ground black pepper, to taste

9 no-boil lasagne noodles

3 ounces aged Cheddar cheese, shredded

Preheat the oven to 350°F.

Heat the oil in a large skillet. Sauté the onion for 3–4 minutes; add the other vegetables and continue cooking for 2–3 minutes. Add the basil, beans, and tomatoes and liquid and heat to boiling; reduce heat and simmer, uncovered, until the sauce is slightly thickened, about 5 minutes. Season to taste with salt and pepper.

Lay 3 lasagne noodles in the bottom of an oiled baking dish. Cover with one-third of the bean mixture. Repeat layers 2 times, finishing with the bean mixture. Sprinkle the cheese on top and bake, uncovered, for 30 minutes until bubbling and golden.

Makes 4 servings.

To balance the meal, serve fresh fruit for dessert.

PER SERVING: 403.5 calories / 19.4 g protein / 57.9 g carbohydrate / 11.3 g fiber / 11.2 g total fat / 5.0 g saturated fat / 22.3 mg cholesterol / 789.1 mg sodium

NUTRITIONAL ANALYSIS PER SERVING

Vitamin A	265.1 RE	Vitamin D	0.3 µg	Thiamin (B-1)	0.2 mg	Vitamin E	0.9 mg
Riboflavin (B-2)	0.3 mg	Calcium	221.0 mg	Niacin	1.6 mg	Iron	3.3 mg
Vitamin B-6	0.3 mg	Phosphorus	249.7 mg	Vitamin B-12	0.2 µg	Magnesium	51.1 mg
Folate (total)	82.4 µg	Zinc	1.6 mg	Vitamin C	70.5 mg	Potassium	563.2 mg

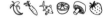

Crispy Vegetable Gratin

This recipe is a super way of serving vegetables to children who do not like them plain.

8 ounces cauliflower, cut into florets

8 ounces broccoli, cut into florets

2 tablespoons butter or margarine

1 tablespoon cornstarch

1 cup milk (skim or part skim is preferable to whole)

1 teaspoon Dijon mustard

3 ounces Cheddar cheese, shredded

Salt and freshly ground black pepper, to taste

2 tablespoons slivered almonds or sesame seeds

Cook the cauliflower and broccoli in boiling water in large saucepan for 5 minutes. Drain.

Melt the butter in a large saucepan. Blend the cornstarch with a little of the milk until smooth. Gradually add the remaining milk. Add to the melted butter and heat to boiling, stirring constantly, until sauce is thickened, about 1 minute; remove from heat. Mix in the mustard and half of the cheese; season to taste with salt and pepper.

Arrange the vegetables in a baking dish and pour the sauce over them. Sprinkle with the remaining cheese and the almonds or sesame seeds. Broil 6 inches from heat source until golden brown.

Makes 4 servings.

To balance the meal, serve with baked or boiled potatoes.

PER SERVING: 226.1 calories / 11.4 g protein / 13.1 g carbohydrate / 3.4 g fiber / 15.4 g total fat / 8.4 g saturated fat / 38.8 mg cholesterol / 265.8 mg sodium

NUTRITIONAL ANALYSIS PER SERVING

Vitamin A	220.6	RE	Vitamin D	0.8 µg	Thiamin (B-1) 0.1 mg	Vitamin E	2.3	mg
Riboflavin (B-2)	0.3	mg	Calcium	282.2 mg	Niacin 0.9 mg	Iron	1.0	mg
Vitamin B-6	0.3	mg	Phosphorus	256.8 mg	Vitamin B-12 0.5 µg	Magnesium	45.8	mg
Folate (total)	76.5	µg	Zinc	1.5 mg	Vitamin C 76.9 mg	Potassium	500.2	mg

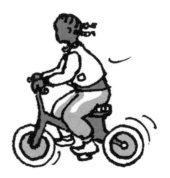

Bean Burritos

These tasty burritos are always popular with children. They include a bean filling that is high in protein, fiber, and iron.

1 tablespoon olive oil

1 small onion, chopped

1 clove garlic, minced

1 tablespoon taco seasoning mix

1 can (15 ounces) pinto or red kidney beans, rinsed and drained

¾ cup thick and/or chunky salsa

4 wheat tortillas (6-inch)

1 cup canned crushed tomatoes with herbs or garlic

2 ounces Cheddar cheese, shredded

Preheat the oven to 350°F.

Heat the oil in a large skillet. Sauté the onion and garlic for 5 minutes. Add the taco seasoning mix, kidney beans, and salsa to the pan. Coarsely mash the beans and cook, uncovered, for 3 minutes, or until the sauce has thickened a little.

Spread one quarter of the mixture over each tortilla. Roll up and place seam-side down in an oiled baking dish. Spoon the tomatoes over the tortillas; bake, loosely covered, until hot through, 20–30 minutes; sprinkle with cheese and bake, uncovered, until cheese is melted, about 5 minutes.

Makes 4 burritos (4 servings).

To balance the meal, serve with a green vegetable or salad.

PER SERVING: 351.7 calories / 13.5 g protein / 44.9 g carbohydrate / 9.5 g fiber / 12.0 g total fat / 3.6 g saturated fat / 14.9 mg cholesterol / 1326.6 mg sodium

NUTRITIONAL ANALYSIS PER SERVING

Vitamin A	119.0 RE	Vitamin D	0.0 µg	Thiamin (B-1) 0.1 mg		Vitamin E	1.6 mg
Riboflavin (B-2) 0.1 mg		Calcium	175.3 mg	Niacin	0.4 mg	Iron	2.4 mg
Vitamin B-6	0.1 mg	Phosphorus	179.0 mg	Vitamin B-12 0.1 µg		Magnesium	35.6 mg
Folate (total)	71.6 µg	Zinc	1.2 mg	Vitamin C	14.4 mg	Potassium	453.6 mg

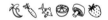

Chickpea Hotpot

This one-pot dish is quick and easy to prepare and makes a perfect midweek supper. Chick-peas are rich in protein, iron, and zinc. Use any variety of canned beans in place of the chick-peas if you wish.

1 tablespoon olive oil

1 small onion, chopped

1 garlic clove, minced

2 small zucchini, sliced

1 teaspoon dried mixed herbs

1 can (14 ounces) chopped tomatoes, undrained

1 can (15 ounces) chickpeas, rinsed and drained

1 cube vegetable bouillon

1½ ounces Cheddar cheese, shredded

Heat the oil in a large saucepan; add the onion and garlic and sauté for 3–4 minutes, until softened. Add the zucchini and cook 2 minutes longer. Add the herbs, tomatoes and liquid, chickpeas, and crumbled bouillon cube; heat to boiling. Reduce heat and simmer, covered, 10 minutes, adding a little water if too thick.

Spoon mixture into a baking dish; sprinkle with cheese. Broil 6 inches from heat source until the cheese is bubbling, 2 to 3 minutes.

Makes 4 servings.

To balance the meal, serve fresh fruit for dessert.

PER SERVING: 248.2 calories / 10.8 g protein / 34.0 g carbohydrate / 7.1 g fiber / 8.7 g total fat / 2.9 g saturated fat / 11.2 mg cholesterol / 973.0 mg sodium

NUTRITIONAL ANALYSIS PER SERVING

Vitamin A	79.9 RE	Vitamin D	0.0 µg	Thiamin (B-1)	0.1 mg	Vitamin E	0.7 mg
Riboflavin (B-2)	0.2 mg	Calcium	141.6 mg	Niacin	0.7 mg	Iron	2.4 mg
Vitamin B-6	0.8 mg	Phosphorus	195.9 mg	Vitamin B-12	0.1 µg	Magnesium	54.0 mg
Folate (total)	106.8 µg	Zinc	1.8 mg	Vitamin C	34.4 mg	Potassium	499.0 mg

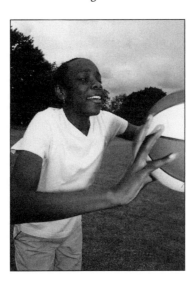

Red Lentil Dahl

Red lentils are a superb source of protein, iron, fiber, and B vitamins.
This mildly spiced dahl will appeal to children.

1 tablespoon canola oil

1 small onion, chopped

1 garlic clove, minced

½ teaspoon ground cumin

1 teaspoon ground coriander

½ teaspoon ground turmeric

6 ounces dried red lentils

3 cups water

Salt and freshly ground black
    pepper, to taste

Heat the oil in a large saucepan and sauté the onion for about 5 minutes. Add the garlic and spices and sauté 2 minutes longer. Add the lentils and water and heat to boiling; reduce heat and simmer, covered, until lentils are tender, about 30 minutes. Season to taste with salt and pepper.

   Makes 4 servings.

To balance the meal, serve with boiled rice and a green vegetable.

PER SERVING: 190.6 calories / 12.4 g protein / 27.8 g carbohydrate / 13.7 g fiber / 4.0 g total fat / 0.3 g saturated fat / 0.0 mg cholesterol / 5.6 mg sodium

NUTRITIONAL ANALYSIS PER SERVING

Vitamin A	1.7 RE	Vitamin D	0.0 µg	Thiamin (B-1)	0.1 mg	Vitamin E	0.9 mg
Riboflavin (B-2)	0.1 mg	Calcium	31.8 mg	Niacin	0.8 mg	Iron	3.2 mg
Vitamin B-6	0.2 mg	Phosphorus	173.4 mg	Vitamin B-12	0.0 µg	Magnesium	37.6 mg
Folate (total)	88.2 µg	Zinc	1.4 mg	Vitamin C	3.8 mg	Potassium	330.4 mg

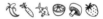

Butter Bean and Leek Supper

This nutritious combination of legumes and vegetables is easy to prepare. You can add other vegetables, such as mushrooms or peppers, to make it a more substantial dish.

2 small leeks, sliced

1 tablespoon olive oil

1 can (14 ounces) chopped
    tomatoes, undrained

1 can (15 ounces) butter
    beans or lima beans,
    rinsed and drained

½ cup vegetable broth

Salt and freshly ground black
    pepper, to taste

Sauté the leeks in olive oil in medium saucepan 5 minutes, or until the leeks are almost soft. Stir in remaining ingredients, except salt and pepper, and heat to boiling. Reduce heat and simmer 10–15 minutes, or until the sauce has thickened. Season to taste with salt and pepper.

   Makes 4 servings.

To balance the meal, serve with new potatoes and grated cheese.

PER SERVING: 155.5 calories / 7.2 g protein / 23.7 g carbohydrate / 5.2 g fiber / 3.9 g total fat / 0.5 g saturated fat / 0.0 mg cholesterol / 651.5 mg sodium

NUTRITIONAL ANALYSIS PER SERVING

Vitamin A	31.9 RE	Vitamin D	0.0 µg	Thiamin (B-1)	0.0 mg	Vitamin E	0.8 mg
Riboflavin (B-2)	0.0 mg	Calcium	71.0 mg	Niacin	0.5 mg	Iron	2.6 mg
Vitamin B-6	0.1 mg	Phosphorus	123.2 mg	Vitamin B-12	0.0 µg	Magnesium	12.5 mg
Folate (total)	28.5 µg	Zinc	0.1 mg	Vitamin C	17.1 mg	Potassium	331.3 mg

Vegetable Korma

Traditional kormas are made with cream. This recipe uses cashews and milk in place of the cream and is a delicious way of introducing children to new flavors. Vary the vegetables according to what you have available.

½ cup milk

1½ ounces cashew pieces

1 tablespoon canola oil

1 small onion, sliced

½ teaspoon each: ground cumin, garam masala*, and turmeric (2 teaspoons mild curry powder can be substituted for the spice combination)

1 garlic clove, minced

4 ounces cauliflower florets

1 small zucchini, sliced

2 ounces mushrooms

1 can (3 ounces) baby corn

Salt, to taste

Heat the milk to boiling in large saucepan; remove from heat and add the cashews. Let stand, covered, 15 minutes; process mixture in blender until smooth and reserve.

Heat the oil in a large saucepan, and sauté the onion for 5 minutes. Add the spices and the garlic and sauté 2 minutes longer. Add the vegetables and reserved cashew mixture; cover and cook over medium heat for 10 minutes or until the vegetables are just tender. Season to taste with the salt.

Makes 4 servings.

To balance the meal, add naan breads (available at Indian markets) or boiled rice.

* Garam masala, an Indian spice blend, is available in the spice section of many supermarkets.

PER SERVING: 146.3 calories / 4.9 g protein / 12.8 g carbohydrate / 2.8 g fiber / 9.3 g total fat / 1.6 g saturated fat / 2.4 mg cholesterol / 77.8 mg sodium

NUTRITIONAL ANALYSIS PER SERVING

Vitamin A	31.6	RE	Vitamin D	0.6	µg	Thiamin (B-1)	0.1	mg	Vitamin E	1.0	mg
Riboflavin (B-2)	0.2	mg	Calcium	71.9	mg	Niacin	1.2	mg	Iron	1.4	mg
Vitamin B-6	0.3	mg	Phosphorus	135.2	mg	Vitamin B-12	0.1	µg	Magnesium	50.0	mg
Folate (total)	46.9	µg	Zinc	1.1	mg	Vitamin C	24.2	mg	Potassium	426.9	mg

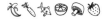

Vegetable Rice Feast

This glorious medley of vegetables and rice is a great way of adding vegetables to children's diets. The peas and pine nuts add protein to the dish.

1 tablespoon olive oil

1 small onion, chopped

1 garlic clove, minced

2 ribs celery, chopped

1 small red or yellow bell pepper, chopped

6 ounces rice (adjust the quantity according to the child's appetite)

1½ cups vegetable broth

4 ounces frozen peas

Salt and freshly ground black pepper, to taste

1 ounce pine nuts or slivered almonds

Heat the oil in a large saucepan, and sauté the onion, garlic, celery, and bell pepper for 5 minutes. Add the rice, and cook, stirring, for another 2–3 minutes. Add the broth and heat to boiling; reduce heat and simmer, covered, 20–25 minutes, until the liquid has been absorbed.

Add the peas during the last 3 minutes of cooking. Season to taste with salt and pepper; serve sprinkled with the pine nuts.

Makes 4 servings.

To balance the meal, add yogurt for dessert.

PER SERVING: 289.3 calories / 6.6 g protein / 46.3 g carbohydrate / 4.1 g fiber / 8.9 g total fat / 0.9 g saturated fat / 0.0 mg cholesterol / 212.8 mg sodium

NUTRITIONAL ANALYSIS PER SERVING

Vitamin A	228.9	RE	Vitamin D	0.0	µg	Thiamin (B-1)	0.3	mg	Vitamin E	1.1	mg
Riboflavin (B-2)	0.1	mg	Calcium	44.9	mg	Niacin	2.9	mg	Iron	3.0	mg
Vitamin B-6	0.3	mg	Phosphorus	252.0	mg	Vitamin B-12	0.0	µg	Magnesium	43.4	mg
Folate (total)	105.7	µg	Zinc	1.3	mg	Vitamin C	62.0	mg	Potassium	369.6	mg

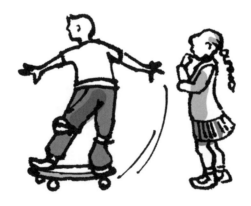

Couscous with Nuts and Vegetables

Couscous is easy to prepare, and children enjoy its soft texture. Mix it with vegetables and nuts to make a delicious, balanced meal.

6 ounces couscous

1½ cups vegetable broth

1 tablespoon olive oil

1 small onion, chopped

1 small red bell pepper, chopped

1 can (3 ounces) baby corn

1 medium carrot, diced

2 ounces dates, chopped (optional)

2 ounces slivered almonds, toasted

Salt and freshly ground black pepper, to taste

Heat the vegetable broth to boiling in medium saucepan; remove from heat and stir in couscous. Let stand, covered, 15 minutes or until all the liquid has been absorbed.

Meanwhile, heat the oil in a skillet and sauté the vegetables for about 7–10 minutes or until crisp-tender.

Fluff the couscous with a fork and stir in the vegetables, dates, and almonds. Season to taste with salt and pepper.

Makes 4 servings.

To balance the meal, add fruit and custard for dessert.

PER SERVING: 313.4 calories / 9.8 g protein / 44.4 g carbohydrate / 6.1 g fiber / 11.2 g total fat / 1.1 g saturated fat / 0.0 mg cholesterol / 236.4 mg sodium

NUTRITIONAL ANALYSIS PER SERVING

Vitamin A	638.4	RE	Vitamin D	0.0	µg	Thiamin (B-1) 0.1 mg	Vitamin E	4.5 mg
Riboflavin (B-2)	0.2	mg	Calcium	69.3	mg	Niacin 2.4 mg	Iron	1.5 mg
Vitamin B-6	0.2	mg	Phosphorus	281.9	mg	Vitamin B-12 0.0 µg	Magnesium	65.8 mg
Folate (total)	23.5	µg	Zinc	1.0	mg	Vitamin C 59.4 mg	Potassium	417.2 mg

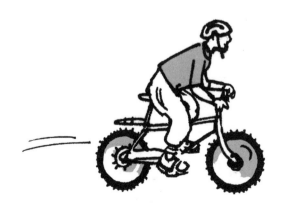

Potato and Cheese Pie

This simple dish of potatoes and cheese is a childhood favorite of mine. My children are equally fond of it. Layer sliced leeks or broccoli florets with the cheese to increase the vegetable content.

1 pound potatoes

2 ounces Cheddar or Swiss cheese, shredded

1 small onion, thinly sliced

2 large tomatoes, sliced

2 eggs

1 cup milk

½ teaspoon salt

⅛ teaspoon freshly ground black pepper

Preheat the oven to 400°F.

Peel and thinly slice the potatoes. Arrange layers of potato, cheese, onion, and tomatoes in a shallow baking dish, finishing with cheese.

Beat the eggs with the milk, salt, and pepper; pour over the potatoes. Cover with foil and bake for 45–60 minutes, until the potatoes are tender; uncover during last 10 minutes to brown top.

Makes 4 servings.

To balance the meal, serve with baked beans and a green vegetable.

PER SERVING: 226.5 calories / 11.4 g protein / 26.3 g carbohydrate / 3.9 g fiber / 8.6 g total fat / 4.6 g saturated fat / 125.5 mg cholesterol / 449.5 mg sodium

NUTRITIONAL ANALYSIS PER SERVING

Vitamin A	148.4 RE	Vitamin D	1.0 µg	Thiamin (B-1)	0.2 mg	Vitamin E	0.7 mg
Riboflavin (B-2)	0.3 mg	Calcium	209.7 mg	Niacin	1.7 mg	Iron	1.4 mg
Vitamin B-6	0.4 mg	Phosphorus	270.2 mg	Vitamin B-12	0.7 µg	Magnesium	47.1 mg
Folate (total)	52.2 µg	Zinc	1.5 mg	Vitamin C	32.0 mg	Potassium	786.7 mg

CHAPTER 16

Salads

Perfect Salad

This salad is an almost perfectly balanced meal. It provides every vitamin and mineral, including calcium from the nuts and yogurt, protein from the red kidney beans and nuts, and carbohydrate from the pasta. To add variety to the salad leaves use field greens, arugula, endive, or baby spinach where available.

4 ounces pasta shells

½ small red bell pepper, chopped

½ small yellow bell pepper, chopped

2 ounces toasted slivered almonds, cashews, or peanuts, chopped

2 ounces raisins

4 ounces rinsed, drained canned red kidney beans

2 small tomatoes, sliced

1 medium apple, sliced

Mixed salad leaves

3 tablespoons plain yogurt

1 tablespoon mayonnaise

Cook the pasta shells in boiling water according to the package directions. Drain and cool.

Mix the pasta with the bell peppers, nuts, raisins, beans, tomatoes, and apple slices.

Spoon over salad leaves on plates.

Mix the yogurt and mayonnaise; spoon on top of salad.

Makes 4 servings.

To balance the meal, add fresh fruit for dessert.

PER SERVING: 325.9 calories / 10.3 g protein / 50.1 g carbohydrate / 6.5 g fiber / 11.0 g total fat / 1.2 g saturated fat / 2.0 mg cholesterol / 134.4 mg sodium

NUTRITIONAL ANALYSIS PER SERVING

Vitamin A	142.5 RE	Vitamin D	0.0 µg	Thiamin (B-1)	0.4 mg	Vitamin E	4.2 mg
Riboflavin (B-2)	0.3 mg	Calcium	80.6 mg	Niacin	3.0 mg	Iron	2.5 mg
Vitamin B-6	0.2 mg	Phosphorus	157.0 mg	Vitamin B-12	0.1 µg	Magnesium	67.5 mg
Folate (total)	105.4 µg	Zinc	0.9 mg	Vitamin C	81.3 mg	Potassium	585.7 mg

Potato Salad

This variation on the American picnic standard is an excellent portable snack or lunch. New potatoes contain twice as much vitamin C as baking potatoes. You can add extra vegetables, such as spring onions and radishes.

1 pound new potatoes or baking potatoes, cut into small chunks

1 tablespoon each chopped mint and parsley

½ cup chopped cucumber

1 tablespoon plain yogurt

1 tablespoon mayonnaise

Salt and freshly ground black pepper, to taste

Cook the potatoes in boiling water for 5–7 minutes until just tender. Drain and cool.

Combine herbs, cucumber, yogurt and mayonnaise; spoon over potatoes and toss. Season to taste with salt and pepper.

Makes 4 servings.

To balance the meal, serve with boiled eggs or cottage cheese and some vegetable crudités.

PER SERVING: 109.1 calories / 2.3 g protein / 18.8 g carbohydrate / 2.9 g fiber / 2.9 g total fat / 0.5 g saturated fat / 1.5 mg cholesterol / 30.0 mg sodium

NUTRITIONAL ANALYSIS PER SERVING

Vitamin A	12.9	RE	Vitamin D	0.0	µg	Thiamin (B-1)	0.1	mg	Vitamin E	0.1	mg
Riboflavin (B-2)	0.1	mg	Calcium	22.2	mg	Niacin	1.2	mg	Iron	0.7	mg
Vitamin B-6	0.3	mg	Phosphorus	80.7	mg	Vitamin B-12	0.0	µg	Magnesium	27.0	mg
Folate (total)	23.9	µg	Zinc	0.4	mg	Vitamin C	24.1	mg	Potassium	498.3	mg

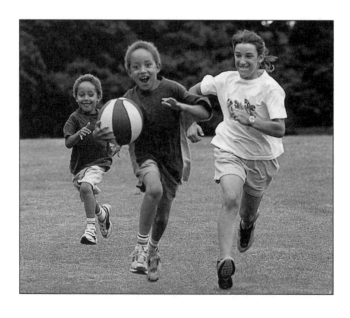

Rice and Corn Salad

This salad is easy to prepare, and the peppers are a great source of vitamin C. The almonds provide protein and calcium.

1½ cups rice (adjust the quantity according to the child's appetite)

1 small red bell pepper, chopped

4 ounces golden or dark raisins

2 ounces blanched almonds, coarsely chopped

1 can (8 ounces) whole kernel corn, drained

Salt and freshly ground black pepper, to taste

Cook the rice according to the package directions; cool.

Combine rice with bell pepper, raisins, almonds, and corn; season to taste with salt and pepper.

Makes 4 servings.

To balance the meal, serve with red kidney beans or hummus.

PER SERVING: 474.9 calories / 10.8 g protein / 93.2 g carbohydrate / 5.2 g fiber / 8.4 g total fat / 0.8 g saturated fat / 0.0 mg cholesterol / 132.8 mg sodium

NUTRITIONAL ANALYSIS PER SERVING

Vitamin A	179.9 RE	Vitamin D	0.0 µg	Thiamin (B-1)	0.4 mg	Vitamin E	4.1 mg
Riboflavin (B-2)	0.2 mg	Calcium	70.0 mg	Niacin	4.7 mg	Iron	4.5 mg
Vitamin B-6	0.3 mg	Phosphorus	221.0 mg	Vitamin B-12	0.0 µg	Magnesium	81.2 mg
Folate (total)	150.4 µg	Zinc	1.6 mg	Vitamin C	62.3 mg	Potassium	558.0 mg

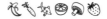

Coleslaw

Children love the crunchiness of shredded cabbage combined with the smooth creaminess of mayonnaise. Raw cabbage is packed with vitamin C, and, though mayonnaise is high in fat, it's mostly the healthy unsaturated kind. Add any of the optional ingredients listed below to the basic recipe–it's a great way of getting your children to eat extra raw vegetables.

4 cups finely shredded green or red cabbage

1 large carrot, peeled and grated

¼ to ½ cup low-fat mayonnaise

Salt and freshly ground black pepper, to taste

Place the cabbage and carrot in a large bowl and stir in mayonnaise. Season to taste with salt and pepper.

Note: Add any of the following ingredients to the salad, if you want: chopped fresh parsley or chives, pineapple chunks, chopped onions or green onions, chopped peppers, red cabbage, chopped broccoli, chopped cauliflower, raisins, cashews, beets, sunflower seeds, toasted pumpkin seeds, grated apple, celery, radicchio, etc.

Makes 4 servings.

PER SERVING: 70.5 calories / 1.1 g protein / 8.0 g carbohydrate / 2.0 g fiber / 4.1 g total fat / 0.5 g saturated fat / 5.0 mg cholesterol / 116.3 mg sodium

NUTRITIONAL ANALYSIS PER SERVING

Vitamin A	434.9 RE	Vitamin D	0.2 µg	Thiamin (B-1)	0.1 mg	Vitamin E	0.5 mg
Riboflavin (B-2)	0.0 mg	Calcium	37.2 mg	Niacin	0.4 mg	Iron	0.5 mg
Vitamin B-6	0.1 mg	Phosphorus	23.9 mg	Vitamin B-12	0.0 µg	Magnesium	12.7 mg
Folate (total)	24.5 µg	Zinc	0.2 mg	Vitamin C	32.1 mg	Potassium	230.0 mg

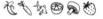

Salad Dressings

Most children reach for commercial salad dressings when confronted with raw salads. However, most store-bought salad dressings are high in salt and contain artificial additives. Here are some quick and healthy alternatives that require no or very little preparation.

- A drizzle of balsamic vinegar
- A squeeze of lemon juice
- Plain yogurt by itself, or mixed with a squeeze of lemon juice and chopped fresh parsley

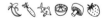

Easy Vinaigrette Dressing

3 tablespoons olive oil

1 tablespoon white or red wine vinegar, or lemon juice

1–2 tablespoons chopped fresh herbs, such as thyme, oregano, basil, marjoram, or parsley (optional)

Pinch of sugar

Pinch of salt

Pinch of freshly ground black pepper

Place the ingredients in a screw-top jar, and shake well to combine.

Use as a dressing for leafy salads, cucumber salad, and bean salads.

Makes 2 servings.

PER SERVING: 181.6 calories / 0.0 g protein / 0.0 g carbohydrate / 0.0 g fiber / 20.3 g total fat / 2.7 g saturated fat / 0.0 mg cholesterol / 1.0 mg sodium

NUTRITIONAL ANALYSIS PER SERVING

Vitamin A	0.0 RE	Vitamin D	0.0 µg	Thiamin (B-1)	0.0 mg	Vitamin E	2.5 mg
Riboflavin (B-2)	0.0 mg	Calcium	0.8 mg	Niacin	0.0 mg	Iron	0.2 mg
Vitamin B-6	0.0 mg	Phosphorus	0.8 mg	Vitamin B-12	0.0 µg	Magnesium	0.0 mg
Folate (total)	0.0 µg	Zinc	0.0 mg	Vitamin C	0.0 mg	Potassium	6.2 mg

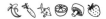

Herb Dressing

¼ cup cider vinegar

2 tablespoons orange juice

1 tablespoon olive oil

1 garlic clove, crushed

1 tablespoon chopped fresh parsley or oregano

Place the ingredients in a screw-top jar, and shake well to combine.

Use as a dressing for lettuce and leafy salads, coleslaw, or with cooked green vegetables, such as broccoli and green beans.

Makes 4 servings.

PER SERVING: 36.9 calories / 0.1 g protein / 2.0 g carbohydrate / 0.1 g fiber / 3.4 g total fat / 0.5 g saturated fat / 0.0 mg cholesterol / 1.0 mg sodium

NUTRITIONAL ANALYSIS PER SERVING

Vitamin A	6.5 RE	Vitamin D	0.0 µg	Thiamin (B-1)	0.0 mg	Vitamin E	0.4 mg
Riboflavin (B-2)	0.0 mg	Calcium	4.5 mg	Niacin	0.0 mg	Iron	0.2 mg
Vitamin B-6	0.0 mg	Phosphorus	4.4 mg	Vitamin B-12	0.0 µg	Magnesium	4.8 mg
Folate (total)	3.8 µg	Zinc	0.0 mg	Vitamin C	5.4 mg	Potassium	38.8 mg

CHAPTER 17

ﾠ🌶🥕🍅🍄🍓

Super Soups

Potato Soup

This is an ideal main-meal soup as it is rich in energy-giving carbohydrate; additionally, the milk provides protein and calcium. Sweet potatoes provide beta-carotene and omega-3 fatty acids, essential for brain development.

To balance the meal, add grated cheese; serve fresh fruit for dessert.

2 tablespoons olive oil

1 small onion, chopped

3 medium potatoes, peeled, cut into ½-inch pieces

1 small sweet potato, peeled, cut into ½-inch pieces

2 teaspoons vegetable bouillon crystals or 1 vegetable bouillon cube

1½ cups water

2 cups fat-free milk

Salt and freshly ground black pepper, to taste

Handful of chopped fresh parsley or thyme, if desired

Heat the oil in a large saucepan. Sauté the onion until transparent, about 5 minutes. Add the potatoes; sauté 2 minutes longer.

Add the vegetable bouillon and the water and heat to boiling; reduce heat and simmer, covered, for about 20 minutes, until the potatoes are soft.

Process soup in blender or food processor until smooth; return to saucepan and stir in milk. Season to taste with salt and pepper, and add desired herbs. Cook, uncovered, over medium heat just until hot, about 5 minutes.

Makes 4 servings.

PER SERVING: 250.9 calories / 7.2 g protein / 40.7 g carbohydrate / 3.1 g fiber / 7.0 g total fat / 1.1 g saturated fat / 2.5 mg cholesterol / 320.3 mg sodium

NUTRITIONAL ANALYSIS PER SERVING

Vitamin A	629.1 RE	Vitamin D	1.2 µg	Thiamin (B-1)	0.2 mg	Vitamin E	1.1 mg
Riboflavin (B-2)	0.3 mg	Calcium	174.3 mg	Niacin	1.9 mg	Iron	0.7 mg
Vitamin B-6	0.5 mg	Phosphorus	204.1 mg	Vitamin B-12	0.6 µg	Magnesium	53.7 mg
Folate (total)	25.1 µg	Zinc	1.0 mg	Vitamin C	17.3 mg	Potassium	793.2 mg

Real Tomato Soup

Tomato soup is a firm favorite with children. It's also a great way of hiding extra vegetables, such as carrots and red peppers. This soup is packed with vitamin C, beta-carotene, and the powerful antioxidant lycopene.

1 small onion, chopped

2 tablespoons olive oil

1 large carrot, grated

1 small red bell pepper, chopped

1 large potato, peeled and cubed

2 garlic cloves, minced

2 teaspoons vegetable bouillon crystals, or 1 vegetable bouillon cube

1 can (14 ounces) chopped tomatoes, undrained

2½ cups water

1 teaspoon sugar

Salt and freshly ground black pepper, to taste

Sauté the onion in the oil for 2–3 minutes in a large saucepan. Add the carrot, red pepper, potato, and garlic, and sauté 5 minutes longer. Add the vegetable bouillon, tomatoes and liquid, water, and sugar and heat to boiling; reduce heat and simmer, covered, for about 20 minutes, or until the vegetables are tender.

Process soup in blender or food processor until smooth; season to taste with salt and pepper.

Makes 4 servings.

To balance the meal, serve with grated cheese and crusty whole-grain bread.

PER SERVING: 148.3 calories / 3.0 g protein / 19.4 g carbohydrate / 3.0 g fiber / 7.3 g total fat / 1.0 g saturated fat / 0.0 mg cholesterol / 467.6 mg sodium

NUTRITIONAL ANALYSIS PER SERVING

Vitamin A	613.5 RE	Vitamin D	0.0 µg	Thiamin (B-1)	0.1 mg	Vitamin E	1.2 mg
Riboflavin (B-2)	0.1 mg	Calcium	26.7 mg	Niacin	1.0 mg	Iron	0.9 mg
Vitamin B-6	0.3 mg	Phosphorus	42.3 mg	Vitamin B-12	0.0 µg	Magnesium	18.8 mg
Folate (total)	17.0 µg	Zinc	0.3 mg	Vitamin C	76.4 mg	Potassium	346.1 mg

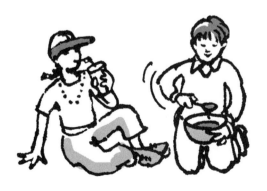

Broccoli and Cheese Soup

This simple soup makes a nutritionally complete meal and is an ingenious way to get children to eat broccoli. It is rich in protein, fiber, vitamin C, and complex carbohydrate.

1 onion, chopped

10 ounces broccoli florets

1½ cups vegetable broth

1½ cups fat-free milk

2 ounces aged Cheddar cheese, shredded

Pinch of freshly grated nutmeg (optional)

Salt and freshly ground black pepper, to taste

Place the onion, broccoli, and vegetable broth in a saucepan. Heat to boiling; reduce heat and simmer, covered, about 15 minutes, or until the vegetables are tender.

Process soup in blender or food processor until smooth; return to the saucepan and add milk. Cook, uncovered, over medium heat until hot, about 5 minutes. Add Cheddar cheese, stirring until it melts. Season to taste with nutmeg, salt, and pepper.

Makes 4 servings.

To balance the meal, serve with crusty whole-grain rolls.

PER SERVING: 132.8 calories / 9.0 g protein / 12.9 g carbohydrate / 2.5 g fiber / 5.0 g total fat / 3.1 g saturated fat / 16.7 mg cholesterol / 317.2 mg sodium

NUTRITIONAL ANALYSIS PER SERVING

Vitamin A	176.4	RE	Vitamin D	0.9	µg	Thiamin (B-1)	0.1	mg	Vitamin E	0.2	mg
Riboflavin (B-2)	0.2	mg	Calcium	247.9	mg	Niacin	0.1	mg	Iron	0.6	mg
Vitamin B-6	0.1	mg	Phosphorus	294.7	mg	Vitamin B-12	0.6	µg	Magnesium	16.8	mg
Folate (total)	12.4	µg	Zinc	0.9	mg	Vitamin C	27.7	mg	Potassium	289.1	mg

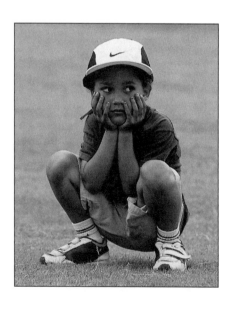

Butternut Squash Soup

This is my children's favorite soup. Butternut squash is very rich in beta-carotene and makes a wonderful soup. Its subtle sweetness appeals to children. You can substitute pumpkin or other varieties of squash for the butternut squash if you wish.

1 small onion, chopped

2 tablespoons olive oil

1 pound butternut squash, peeled and chopped

1 large carrot, sliced

1 medium potato, peeled and chopped

2 teaspoons vegetable bouillon powder or 1 vegetable bouillon cube

3 cups water

1 teaspoon grated fresh ginger, or ½ teaspoon ground ginger

Salt and freshly ground black pepper, to taste

Sauté the onion in the olive oil in large saucepan for about 5 minutes, or until transparent. Add the butternut squash, carrot, and potato, and sauté 2–3 minutes longer. Add the vegetable bouillon, water, and ginger and heat to boiling; reduce heat and simmer, covered until the vegetables are tender, about 15 minutes.

Process the soup in blender or food processor until smooth; season to taste with salt and pepper.

Makes 4 servings.

To balance the meal, serve with grated cheese and whole-grain bread.

PER SERVING: 169.0 calories / 2.6 g protein / 26.3 g carbohydrate / 3.8 g fiber / 7.0 g total fat / 1.0 g saturated fat / 0.0 mg cholesterol / 265.5 mg sodium

NUTRITIONAL ANALYSIS PER SERVING

Vitamin A	1,134.8 RE	Vitamin D	0.0 µg	Thiamin (B-1)	0.1 mg	Vitamin E	1.0 mg
Riboflavin (B-2)	0.1 mg	Calcium	64.5 mg	Niacin	2.0 mg	Iron	1.4 mg
Vitamin B-6	0.4 mg	Phosphorus	79.7 mg	Vitamin B-12	0.0 µg	Magnesium	51.9 mg
Folate (total)	44.2 µg	Zinc	0.4 mg	Vitamin C	24.5 mg	Potassium	702.4 mg

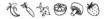

Carrot Soup

This soup is inexpensive and simple to make. It is also packed with the antioxidant beta-carotene.

1 small onion, chopped

1 clove of garlic, minced

2 tablespoons olive oil

1 pound carrots, sliced

3 cups vegetable broth

Salt and freshly ground black pepper, to taste

1–2 tablespoons chopped fresh cilantro (optional)

Sauté the onion and garlic in the olive oil in large saucepan until tender, about 5 minutes. Add the carrots, and sauté 2 minutes longer. Add the broth and heat to boiling; reduce heat and simmer, covered, 15 minutes or until the carrots are tender. Season to taste with the salt and pepper, and add the cilantro. Process the soup in blender or food processor until smooth.
Makes 4 servings.

To balance the meal, add a swirl of plain yogurt or grated cheese and serve with crusty whole-grain rolls.

PER SERVING: 141.3 calories / 2.1 g protein / 17.6 g carbohydrate / 4.3 g fiber / 7.4 g total fat / 1.0 g saturated fat / 0.0 mg cholesterol / 424.4 mg sodium

NUTRITIONAL ANALYSIS PER SERVING

Vitamin A	2,945.9	RE	Vitamin D	0.0	µg	Thiamin (B-1)	0.1	mg	Vitamin E	1.4	mg
Riboflavin (B-2)	0.1	mg	Calcium	59.9	mg	Niacin	1.1	mg	Iron	0.7	mg
Vitamin B-6	0.2	mg	Phosphorus	292.0	mg	Vitamin B-12	0.0	µg	Magnesium	16.5	mg
Folate (total)	22.5	µg	Zinc	0.3	mg	Vitamin C	7.0	mg	Potassium	590.0	mg

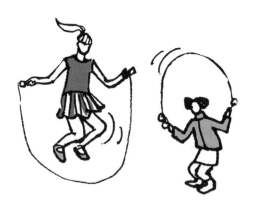

Vegetable and Pasta Soup

This soup is ideal for hiding vegetables your children may not normally choose to eat on their own. Vary the vegetables according to what you have available.

1 small onion, chopped

1 garlic clove, minced

1 small red bell pepper, chopped

2 tablespoons olive oil

2 large carrots, chopped

4 ounces cauliflower florets

2 medium potatoes, peeled and cubed

3½ cups vegetable broth

1 can (14 ounces) chopped tomatoes, undrained

3 ounces small pasta shapes

4 ounces frozen peas

Salt and freshly ground black pepper, to taste

Sauté the onion, garlic, and red pepper in the olive oil in large saucepan for 5 minutes. Add carrots, cauliflower, and potatoes and cook 2 minutes longer. Add the vegetable broth and tomatoes and liquid; heat to boiling. Reduce heat and simmer, covered, 20 minutes, adding the pasta and frozen peas 10 minutes before the end of the cooking time. Season to taste with salt and pepper.

To balance the meal, add grated cheese.

Tip: For a chunky thick soup, purée half the vegetables and broth before the pasta and peas are added in blender or food processor; stir into soup in the pan.

Makes 4–6 servings.

PER SERVING: 305.3 calories / 9.3 g protein / 49.7 g carbohydrate / 8.4 g fiber / 8.3 g total fat / 1.0 g saturated fat / 0.0 mg cholesterol / 667.5 mg sodium

NUTRITIONAL ANALYSIS PER SERVING

Vitamin A	1,149.0 RE	Vitamin D	0.0 µg	Thiamin (B-1)	0.4 mg	Vitamin E	1.3 mg
Riboflavin (B-2)	0.2 mg	Calcium	60.4 mg	Niacin	3.0 mg	Iron	2.6 mg
Vitamin B-6	0.4 mg	Phosphorus	385.9 mg	Vitamin B-12	0.0 µg	Magnesium	34.3 mg
Folate (total)	93.4 µg	Zinc	0.6 mg	Vitamin C	99.6 mg	Potassium	795.6 mg

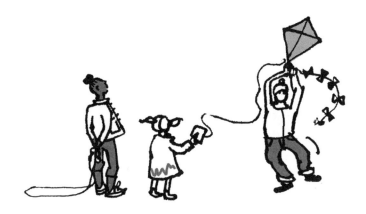

CHAPTER 18

🍌🥕⭐🍅🥜🍓

Fast Food

Homemade Chicken Nuggets

These homemade chicken nuggets are far healthier than the frozen and takeout versions. The wheat germ used for the coating provides essential B vitamins (thiamin and niacin), iron, and zinc. They are baked rather than fried, reducing the fat content and the need for artificial flavor enhancers.

To balance the meal, serve with Oven Potato Wedges (page 182), carrots, and peas.

1 pound boneless, skinless chicken breast

3 tablespoons wheat germ

½ teaspoon salt

½ teaspoon garlic powder

⅛ teaspoon freshly ground black pepper

¼ cup water

1 egg white

Preheat the oven to 400°F.

Cut the chicken breast into ½-inch pieces. Combine the wheat germ, salt, garlic powder, and pepper in a large plastic bag.

Combine the water and egg white in a bowl. Dip the chicken pieces into the egg mixture, and then place in the plastic bag; shake until the chicken is thoroughly coated. Place the coated chicken pieces in an oiled baking pan. Bake, uncovered, 15 to 20 minutes, or until tender and golden brown, turning once after 10 minutes.

Makes 4 servings.

PER SERVING: 148.5 calories / 28.7 g protein / 2.6 g carbohydrate / 0.8 g fiber / 1.7 g total fat / 0.4 g saturated fat / 65.7 mg cholesterol / 363.6 mg sodium

NUTRITIONAL ANALYSIS PER SERVING

Vitamin A	5.7 RE	Vitamin D	0.0 µg	Thiamin (B-1)	0.2 mg	Vitamin E	1.4 mg
Riboflavin (B-2)	0.2 mg	Calcium	15.8 mg	Niacin	10.4 mg	Iron	1.1 mg
Vitamin B-6	0.5 mg	Phosphorus	235.7 mg	Vitamin B-12	0.3 µg	Magnesium	40.4 mg
Folate (total)	22.1 µg	Zinc	1.7 mg	Vitamin C	1.5 mg	Potassium	302.2 mg

Chicken Burgers

These are a healthy alternative to beef burgers due to their lower fat content.

1 small onion, finely
  chopped

1 rib celery, finely chopped

1 clove garlic, minced

2 tablespoons olive oil

1 pound boneless, skinless
  chicken breasts, cut into
  ½-inch pieces

2 tablespoons chopped
  parsley

½ cup fresh bread crumbs

½ teaspoon salt

⅛ teaspoon freshly ground
  black pepper

1 egg yolk

Flour for coating

Sauté the onion, celery, and garlic in the olive oil in medium skillet until onion is tender, about 5 minutes. Meanwhile mince or finely chop the chicken in a food processor. Combine the onion mixture, chicken, and remaining ingredients (except the flour).

Form into 4 burgers, roll them in the flour to coat and cook over medium heat in greased medium skillet until browned and cooked, 5–6 minutes each side.

Makes 4 burgers (4 servings).

To balance the meal, add a whole-grain bun, shredded lettuce, sliced tomatoes, sliced onion, and a little salsa or relish.

PER SERVING: 232.0 calories / 28.6 g protein / 6.4 g carbohydrate / 0.8 g fiber / 9.6 g total fat / 1.7 g saturated fat / 118.6 mg cholesterol / 415.7 mg sodium

NUTRITIONAL ANALYSIS PER SERVING

Vitamin A	40.2 RE	Vitamin D	0.2 µg	Thiamin (B-1)	0.1 mg	Vitamin E	1.3 mg
Riboflavin (B-2)	0.2 mg	Calcium	41.5 mg	Niacin	10.5 mg	Iron	1.4 mg
Vitamin B-6	0.6 mg	Phosphorus	219.4 mg	Vitamin B-12	0.4 µg	Magnesium	31.7 mg
Folate (total)	26.6 µg	Zinc	1.2 mg	Vitamin C	5.9 mg	Potassium	333.8 mg

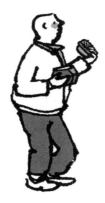

Spicy Bean Burgers

This is a great vegetarian treat that even my children's nonvegetarian friends enjoy. The beans are a good source of protein, iron, and B vitamins, but you can use other beans, such as pinto beans or black beans, instead. You can hide lots of vegetables in the burgers, too.

1 tablespoon olive oil

1 small onion, chopped

1 clove of garlic, minced

1 rib celery, chopped

1 small carrot, finely grated

1 small green bell pepper, chopped

½ teaspoon ground cumin

½ teaspoon ground coriander

1 tablespoon chopped cilantro (optional)

2 cans (15 ounces each) red kidney beans, rinsed and drained, mashed

1 tablespoon tomato purée

1 egg

½ cup dry unseasoned bread crumbs

2 ounces Cheddar cheese, grated

½ teaspoon salt

⅛ teaspoon freshly ground black pepper

Preheat oven to 400°F.

Heat the oil in a medium skillet and sauté the onion for 3–4 minutes until transparent. Add the garlic, celery, carrot, green pepper, and spices, and cook for 5 minutes longer. Add the mashed beans, tomato purée, cheese, bread crumbs, egg, salt, and pepper. Mix, then shape into 8 small or 4 large burgers.

Place burgers in an oiled baking pan. Bake 25 minutes, until browned and crisp.

Makes 8 small or 4 large burgers (4 servings).

To balance the meal, add a whole-grain bun, lettuce, sliced tomatoes, onion, and salsa.

PER SERVING: 369.3 calories / 19.0 g protein / 49.8 g carbohydrate / 16.0 g fiber / 11.0 g total fat / 4.1 g saturated fat / 67.8 mg cholesterol / 1242.2 mg sodium

NUTRITIONAL ANALYSIS PER SERVING

Vitamin A	518.9 RE	Vitamin D	0.2 µg	Thiamin (B-1)	0.4 mg	Vitamin E	1.2 mg
Riboflavin (B-2)	0.4 mg	Calcium	208.5 mg	Niacin	2.2 mg	Iron	4.0 mg
Vitamin B-6	0.2 mg	Phosphorus	341.0 mg	Vitamin B-12	0.3 µg	Magnesium	79.8 mg
Folate (total)	146.3 µg	Zinc	2.0 mg	Vitamin C	30.0 mg	Potassium	782.4 mg

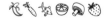

Lean Meat Burgers

These homemade burgers are made with lean ground meat and cooked without extra oil. This means they are low in fat—and you know exactly what's in them!

1 pound extra-lean ground meat (beef, turkey, pork)

½ cup dry unseasoned bread crumbs

3 tablespoons water

1 small onion, chopped

2 tablespoons chopped sage or parsley, or 1 tablespoon dried sage or parsley

½ teaspoon salt

⅛ teaspoon freshly ground black pepper

Mix the ground meat, onion, bread crumbs, water, herbs, salt, and pepper in a bowl. Shape the mixture into 4 large or 8 small burgers. Cook in greased medium skillet over medium heat for 3–4 minutes on each side, or until browned and cooked through. Or, place the burgers in a baking pan and bake at 400°F for 10–15 minutes. Check if the burgers are done by inserting a skewer into the middle of one—there should be no trace of pink, and the juices should run clear.

Makes 4 servings—8 small or 4 large burgers

To balance the meal, add a whole-grain bun, shredded lettuce, sliced tomatoes, relish or salsa, and plenty of salad.

PER SERVING: 308.2 calories / 23.1 g protein / 10.8 g carbohydrate / 0.7 g fiber / 18.4 g total fat / 7.0 g saturated fat / 76.3 mg cholesterol / 464.7 mg sodium

NUTRITIONAL ANALYSIS PER SERVING

Vitamin A	3.8 RE	Vitamin D	0.0 µg	Thiamin (B-1)	0.2 mg	Vitamin E	0.3 mg
Riboflavin (B-2)	0.3 mg	Calcium	45.2 mg	Niacin	5.5 mg	Iron	2.9 mg
Vitamin B-6	0.2 mg	Phosphorus	184.8 mg	Vitamin B-12	1.8 µg	Magnesium	32.1 mg
Folate (total)	22.1 µg	Zinc	4.9 mg	Vitamin C	0.5 mg	Potassium	366.4 mg

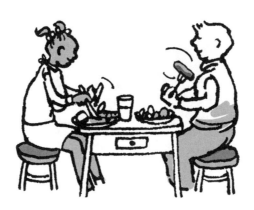

Spicy Lentil Burgers

These tasty burgers are made with red lentils, a terrific source of protein, iron, and fiber. They are oven-baked using only a little oil.

1 tablespoon olive oil

1 small onion, finely chopped

1–2 teaspoons curry powder (adjust according to the child's tastes)

6 ounces dried red lentils

2 cups vegetable stock

1 cup fresh whole-grain bread crumbs

Salt and freshly ground black pepper, to taste

Olive oil

Preheat oven to 400°F.

Heat the olive oil in a large saucepan and sauté the onion until softened. Stir in the curry powder and cook 2 minutes longer. Add the lentils and stock and heat to boiling; reduce heat and simmer, covered, until lentils are tender and stock is absorbed, 20–25 minutes. Cool slightly, then mix in the bread crumbs. Season to taste with salt and pepper.

Shape mixture into 4 large or 8 small burgers. Place in an oiled baking pan and brush lightly with olive oil. Bake for 7–10 minutes, until browned.

Makes 8 small or 4 large burgers (4 servings).

To balance the meal, add a whole-grain bun or baked potato, shredded lettuce, sliced tomatoes, onion, and a little salsa or relish.

PER SERVING: 232.3 calories / 13.7 g protein / 35.4 g carbohydrate / 14.8 g fiber / 4.8 g total fat / 0.7 g saturated fat / 0.1 mg cholesterol / 310.4 mg sodium

NUTRITIONAL ANALYSIS PER SERVING

Vitamin A	52.6 RE	Vitamin D	0.0 µg	Thiamin (B-1)	0.2 mg	Vitamin E	0.8 mg
Riboflavin (B-2)	0.1 mg	Calcium	42.6 mg	Niacin	1.2 mg	Iron	3.8 mg
Vitamin B-6	0.2 mg	Phosphorus	360.3 mg	Vitamin B-12	0.0 µg	Magnesium	49.1 mg
Folate (total)	92.7 µg	Zinc	1.6 mg	Vitamin C	3.5 mg	Potassium	482.0 mg

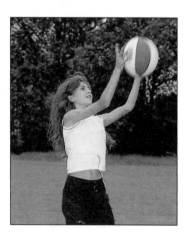

Nut Burgers

These delicious burgers are a real hit with my children. Nuts are a terrific source of essential fats, protein, iron, zinc, and B vitamins. You can substitute other types of nuts, such as almonds, hazelnuts, or peanuts, for the cashews if you wish.

1 small onion, chopped

1 garlic clove, minced

½ small red bell pepper, chopped

1 tablespoon canola oil

1 teaspoon dried mixed herbs

1 tablespoon whole-wheat flour

⅔ cup water

½ vegetable bouillon cube

8 ounces cashews, ground

1 cup fresh whole-grain bread crumbs

Salt and freshly ground black pepper, to taste

Olive oil

Preheat the oven to 400°F.

Sauté the onion, garlic, and red pepper in the oil in medium skillet for 5 minutes until translucent. Add the herbs and flour and cook 2 minutes longer. Stir in the water and bouillon cube, and cook over medium-high heat, stirring, until thickened. Stir in the cashews and bread crumbs; season with salt and pepper to taste. Allow to cool slightly.

Shape mixture into 4–8 burgers and arrange on an oiled baking sheet. Brush lightly with olive oil. Bake 15–20 minutes, until browned.

Makes 4 large or 8 small burgers (4 servings).

To balance the meal, serve with mashed potatoes, carrots, and peas.

PER SERVING: 409.6 calories / 10.3 g protein / 29.4 g carbohydrate / 3.4 g fiber / 30.5 g total fat / 5.6 g saturated fat / 0.0 mg cholesterol / 333.3 mg sodium

NUTRITIONAL ANALYSIS PER SERVING

Vitamin A	85.5 RE	Vitamin D	0.0 µg	Thiamin (B-1)	0.2 mg	Vitamin E	1.4 mg
Riboflavin (B-2)	0.2 mg	Calcium	40.3 mg	Niacin	1.5 mg	Iron	3.9 mg
Vitamin B-6	0.3 mg	Phosphorus	321.3 mg	Vitamin B-12	0.0 µg	Magnesium	165.9 mg
Folate (total)	51.7 µg	Zinc	3.5 mg	Vitamin C	30.3 mg	Potassium	447.4 mg

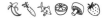

Tomato Salsa

Tomato salsa makes a great accompaniment to tacos, burritos, grilled chicken, and meat or vegetarian burgers. It also enlivens steamed or roasted vegetables, scrambled eggs, and cheese on toast.

2 medium tomatoes, seeded and finely diced

1–2 tablespoons chopped fresh cilantro

1 teaspoon finely chopped fresh jalapeno or serrano chili, or ½ teaspoon chili flakes (adjust according to the child's tastes)

1 small clove garlic, minced

1 tablespoon olive oil

2 green onions, finely chopped

2 tablespoons lemon or lime juice

Combine all the ingredients in a bowl; refrigerate until serving time.

Makes 4 servings.

PER SERVING: 46.7 calories / 0.8 g protein / 3.9 g carbohydrate / 1.0 g fiber / 3.5 g total fat / 0.5 g saturated fat / 0.0 mg cholesterol / 4.6 mg sodium

NUTRITIONAL ANALYSIS PER SERVING

Vitamin A	41.4 RE	Vitamin D	0.0 µg	Thiamin (B-1)	0.0 mg	Vitamin E	0.7 mg
Riboflavin (B-2)	0.0 mg	Calcium	13.6 mg	Niacin	0.4 mg	Iron	0.3 mg
Vitamin B-6	0.0 mg	Phosphorus	19.4 mg	Vitamin B-12	0.0 µg	Magnesium	9.1 mg
Folate (total)	15.5 µg	Zinc	0.1 mg	Vitamin C	13.4 mg	Potassium	180.9 mg

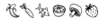

Pizza

Making your own pizzas is easy if you have a bread machine. Alternatively, use the quick pizza-crust recipe (see the recipe that follows); it doesn't require kneading or rising. It's worth making your own tomato sauce, too, as store-bought versions contain quite a lot of salt and have a processed flavor we don't want children to get used to.

1¾ cups all-purpose flour

½ packet fast-rising dry yeast

½ teaspoon salt

1 tablespoon olive oil

¾ cup hot water (120°F)

¾ cup pizza sauce

Pizza toppings (chopped onion, green pepper, tomatoes, mushrooms, shredded mozzarella cheese, etc.)

Mix the flour, yeast, and salt in a large bowl. Make a well in the center and add the oil and half the water. Stir with a wooden spoon, gradually adding enough remaining water to make a soft dough. Knead the dough on a floured surface for about 5 minutes, until smooth and elastic. Place the dough in an oiled bowl, cover with a tea towel, and leave in a warm place for about 1 hour, or until doubled in size.

Punch dough down; knead briefly on floured surface. Roll into a 12-inch circle; place on oiled 12-inch pizza pan and make a rim around the edge. Spread pizza sauce over dough and sprinkle with toppings. Bake at 425°F for 15–20 minutes, or until the crust is golden brown.

Notes: To make the dough with a bread machine, place the ingredients in the container and follow the manufacturer's instructions.

For a thicker crust, let the dough rise for 30 minutes after placing it on the pizza pan.

Makes 1 large pizza (4 servings).

PER SERVING: 251.3 calories / 7.0 g protein / 45.9 g carbohydrate / 3.0 g fiber / 4.4 g total fat / 0.5 g saturated fat / 0.0 mg cholesterol / 434.8 mg sodium

NUTRITIONAL ANALYSIS PER SERVING

Vitamin A	3.9 RE	Vitamin D	0.0 µg	Thiamin (B-1)	0.5 mg	Vitamin E	0.5 mg
Riboflavin (B-2)	0.3 mg	Calcium	18.6 mg	Niacin	3.6 mg	Iron	2.9 mg
Vitamin B-6	0.0 mg	Phosphorus	70.2 mg	Vitamin B-12	0.0 µg	Magnesium	12.9 mg
Folate (total)	120.3 µg	Zinc	0.4 mg	Vitamin C	10.4 mg	Potassium	75.9 mg

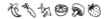

Quick Pizza

1¾ cups self-rising flour

1 teaspoon baking powder

½ teaspoon salt

3 tablespoons butter or margarine, cold

⅔ cup fat-free milk

¾ cup pizza sauce

Pizza toppings (chopped onion, green pepper, tomatoes, mushrooms, shredded mozzarella cheese, etc.)

Mix the flour, baking powder, and salt in a bowl. Using a pastry blender or two dinner knives, cut in the butter or margarine until the mixture resembles coarse crumbs. Add the milk, quickly mixing with a fork, just until the mixture comes together.

Roll the dough on floured surface into a 12-inch circle and place on a 12-inch pizza pan; make rim around the edge. Spread dough with pizza sauce and sprinkle with toppings. Bake at 425°F for 15 minutes, or until crust is golden brown.

Makes 1 large pizza (4 servings).

PER SERVING: 304.3 calories / 7.9 g protein / 46.8 g carbohydrate / 2.9 g fiber / 9.6 g total fat / 5.6 g saturated fat / 23.7 mg cholesterol / 1328.1 mg sodium

NUTRITIONAL ANALYSIS PER SERVING

Vitamin A	82.2 RE	Vitamin D	0.6 µg	Thiamin (B-1)	0.4 mg	Vitamin E	0.2 mg
Riboflavin (B-2)	0.3 mg	Calcium	315.9 mg	Niacin	3.2 mg	Iron	2.9 mg
Vitamin B-6	0.0 mg	Phosphorus	394.4 mg	Vitamin B-12	0.2 µg	Magnesium	15.4 mg
Folate (total)	109.6 µg	Zinc	0.5 mg	Vitamin C	10.4 mg	Potassium	134.4 mg

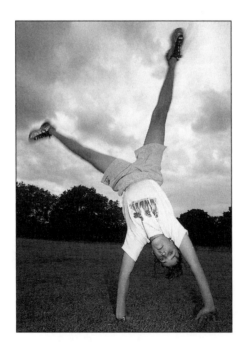

Cheese and Tomato Pizza

This is a great opportunity to add extra vegetables to your children's diet. Add any combination of the following: sliced tomatoes, halved cherry tomatoes, sliced bell peppers, sliced mushrooms, whole kernel corn, chopped onion, olives, sliced zucchini, flaked tuna, spinach leaves, broccoli florets, pineapple chunks, various cheeses, cooked turkey or chicken, etc.

1 small onion, finely chopped

1 garlic clove, minced

1 tablespoon olive oil

1 cup tomato puree, or 1 can (14 ounces) chopped tomatoes, drained

1 tablespoon tomato paste

1 teaspoon dried basil

½ teaspoon sugar

Pinch of salt and freshly ground black pepper

12-inch pizza crust (home-made or purchased)

4 ounces shredded mozzarella or Cheddar cheese

Sauté the onion and garlic in the olive oil in large saucepan for 5 minutes, or until translucent. Add the tomato puree, tomato paste, basil, sugar, salt, and pepper; heat to boiling. Reduce heat and simmer, uncovered, 5–10 minutes, or until the sauce has thickened a little.

Spread the sauce on the pizza crust and sprinkle with cheese. Bake at 450°F for 15–20 minutes, until the cheese is bubbling and crust is golden brown.

***Note:* Alternative pizza crusts:** toasted split bagels or English muffins, focaccia, ciabatta, whole-grain or white pita bread, French bread, etc.

Makes 1 large pizza (4 servings).

PER SERVING: 450.9 calories / 21.6 g protein / 58.8 g carbohydrate / 1.2 g fiber / 16.0 g total fat / 4.0 g saturated fat / 23.9 mg cholesterol / 862.2 mg sodium

NUTRITIONAL ANALYSIS PER SERVING

Vitamin A	204.4 RE	Vitamin D	0.0 µg	Thiamin (B-1)	0.0 mg	Vitamin E	0.8 mg
Riboflavin (B-2)	0.0 mg	Calcium	387.1 mg	Niacin	1.1 mg	Iron	1.2 mg
Vitamin B-6	0.1 mg	Phosphorus	1,376.2 mg	Vitamin B-12	0.0 µg	Magnesium	3.1 mg
Folate (total)	6.7 µg	Zinc	0.1 mg	Vitamin C	12.1 mg	Potassium	185.0 mg

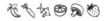

Baked Potatoes

Baked potatoes are nutritious, delicious, and simple to prepare. They provide complex carbohydrates, B vitamins, vitamin C, iron, and fiber.

4 medium or large potatoes

Here's how to bake the perfect potato:

Wash the potatoes, and pierce the skin with a fork.

Bake directly on the oven shelf at 425°F for about 1 to 1¼ hours, or until the flesh is very tender.

Note: For a crispy skin, rub potatoes lightly with a little olive oil and salt.

Toppings for baked potatoes: baked beans, Cheddar cheese, mozzarella cheese, plain yogurt, salsa, stir-fried vegetables, chicken mixed with a little mayonnaise, Hummus (see page 193), low-fat cottage cheese, shrimp salad, ratatouille, Red Lentil Dahl (see page 154), tuna salad, grilled mushrooms, Chili con Carne (see page 141), scrambled egg and tomato, corn, Bolognese sauce (see Pasta Turkey Bolognese on page 133), Vegetarian Spaghetti Bolognese (see page 145), Vegetable Korma (see page 155).

Makes 4 servings.

PER SERVING: 187.9 calories / 5.1 g protein / 42.7 g carbohydrate / 4.4 g fiber / 0.3 g total fat / 0.1 g saturated fat / 0.0 mg cholesterol / 20.2 mg sodium

NUTRITIONAL ANALYSIS PER SERVING

Vitamin A	0.0 RE	Vitamin D	0.0 µg	Thiamin (B-1)	0.1 mg	Vitamin E	0.1 mg
Riboflavin (B-2)	0.1 mg	Calcium	30.3 mg	Niacin	2.8 mg	Iron	2.2 mg
Vitamin B-6	0.6 mg	Phosphorus	141.4 mg	Vitamin B-12	0.0 µg	Magnesium	56.6 mg
Folate (total)	56.6 µg	Zinc	0.7 mg	Vitamin C	19.4 mg	Potassium	1,080.7 mg

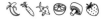

Mighty Root Mash

The rutabaga and parsnips impart a subtle sweetness, which children love. They also add extra vitamins to the dish. Extra milk is used in place of the traditional butter to create a soft consistency.

1 pound potatoes, peeled and cubed

4 ounces rutabaga, peeled and cubed

1 small parsnip, peeled and cubed

¾ cup milk, warm

Salt and freshly ground black pepper, to taste

Cook the potato, rutabaga, and parsnip in boiling water, covered in large saucepan, for 15–20 minutes, or until tender. Drain. Mash vegetables with the milk. Season to taste with salt and pepper.

Makes 4 servings.

To balance the meal, serve with Chicken Burgers (page 171) or Spicy Bean Burgers (page 172) and a green vegetable.

PER SERVING: 124.9 calories / 4.0 g protein / 25.2 g carbohydrate / 4.2 g fiber / 1.1 g total fat / 0.6 g saturated fat / 3.7 mg cholesterol / 32.9 mg sodium

NUTRITIONAL ANALYSIS PER SERVING

Vitamin A	33.7 RE	Vitamin D	0.5 µg	Thiamin (B-1)	0.1 mg	Vitamin E	0.1 mg
Riboflavin (B-2)	0.1 mg	Calcium	83.0 mg	Niacin	1.6 mg	Iron	0.8 mg
Vitamin B-6	0.3 mg	Phosphorus	141.5 mg	Vitamin B-12	0.2 µg	Magnesium	40.2 mg
Folate (total)	39.7 µg	Zinc	0.7 mg	Vitamin C	32.3 mg	Potassium	687.7 mg

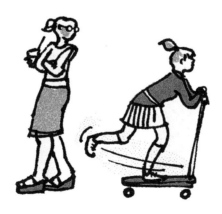

Oven Potato Wedges

These are a real treat for my children. These oven-baked wedges are healthier than fries: they are lower in fat and, with the skins left on, retain much of their vitamin C.

4 medium potatoes (adjust the quantity according to the child's appetite)

4 teaspoons canola or olive oil

Optional: garlic powder, Parmesan cheese, chili powder

Salt and freshly ground black pepper, to taste

Preheat the oven to 400°F.

Cut each potato lengthwise in half; then cut each half into 4 wedges. Place in a baking pan and brush lightly with oil. Bake, uncovered for 35–40 minutes, turning occasionally, until the potatoes are soft inside and golden brown on the outside. Sprinkle on one of the optional ingredients 5 minutes before the end of cooking. Sprinkle lightly with salt and pepper.

To balance the meal, serve with baked beans or scrambled eggs and a green vegetable.

Makes 4 servings.

PER SERVING: 198.8 calories / 3.8 g protein / 35.6 g carbohydrate / 5.4 g fiber / 4.8 g total fat / 0.4 g saturated fat / 0.0 mg cholesterol / 13.6 mg sodium

NUTRITIONAL ANALYSIS PER SERVING

Vitamin A	0.0 RE	Vitamin D	0.0 µg	Thiamin (B-1)	0.2 mg	Vitamin E	1.0 mg
Riboflavin (B-2)	0.1 mg	Calcium	20.4 mg	Niacin	2.4 mg	Iron	1.2 mg
Vitamin B-6	0.5 mg	Phosphorus	140.6 mg	Vitamin B-12	0.0 µg	Magnesium	47.6 mg
Folate (total)	40.8 µg	Zinc	0.7 mg	Vitamin C	44.7 mg	Potassium	923.1 mg

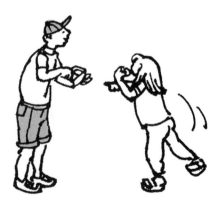

Potato Tacos

These tacos are easy to assemble and very nutritious, too. The beans supply protein, iron, B vitamins, and fiber and make a tasty partner to the baked potatoes.

4 medium potatoes, scrubbed

Olive oil

Salt

¾ cup canned refried beans

¼ cup mild taco sauce or salsa

4 ounces Cheddar cheese, shredded

¼ cup plain low-fat yogurt

Shredded iceberg lettuce

1 small tomato, finely chopped

Preheat the oven to 400°F.

Pierce potatoes with a fork. Rub with a little oil and salt. Bake on oven rack 1 hour, or until tender. Split the cooked potato and puff it up.

Heat the refried beans. Spoon the beans and sauce on top of the potato. Top with the grated cheese and yogurt. Sprinkle the lettuce and tomato on top.

Makes 4 servings.

To balance the meal, add pepper strips and cucumber slices.

PER SERVING: 359.8 calories / 15.4 g protein / 52.7 g carbohydrate / 7.1 g fiber / 10.1 g total fat / 6.2 g saturated fat / 30.7 mg cholesterol / 507.3 mg sodium

NUTRITIONAL ANALYSIS PER SERVING

Vitamin A	100.3 RE	Vitamin D	0.1 µg	Thiamin (B-1)	0.2 mg	Vitamin E	0.3 mg
Riboflavin (B-2)	0.3 mg	Calcium	280.8 mg	Niacin	3.2 mg	Iron	3.1 mg
Vitamin B-6	0.7 mg	Phosphorus	316.0 mg	Vitamin B-12	0.3 µg	Magnesium	70.5 mg
Folate (total)	68.0 µg	Zinc	1.8 mg	Vitamin C	23.4 mg	Potassium	1,340.9 mg

CHAPTER 19

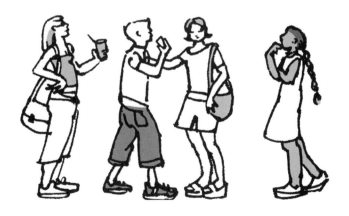

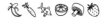

And to Finish

Raspberry Fool

Raspberries are full of vitamin C, and the yogurt provides protein and calcium. You may substitute other seasonal fruits such as strawberries, blackberries, or, in the winter, mango or applesauce.

8 ounces fresh raspberries

8 ounces low-fat vanilla
   yogurt

1 tablespoon honey

Mash the raspberries lightly with a fork.
   Mix with the yogurt and honey. Spoon into 4 bowls.
   Makes 4 servings.

PER SERVING: 93.6 calories / 3.5 g protein / 18.9 g carbohydrate / 3.7 g fiber / 1.1 g total fat / 0.5 g saturated fat / 2.8 mg cholesterol / 38.2 mg sodium

NUTRITIONAL ANALYSIS PER SERVING

Vitamin A	14.7	RE	Vitamin D	0.0 µg	Thiamin (B-1)	0.0 mg	Vitamin E	0.3 mg
Riboflavin (B-2)	0.1	mg	Calcium	111.4 mg	Niacin	0.4 mg	Iron	0.5 mg
Vitamin B-6	0.1	mg	Phosphorus	93.2 mg	Vitamin B-12	0.3 µg	Magnesium	21.7 mg
Folate (total)	18.2	µg	Zinc	0.7 mg	Vitamin C	15.3 mg	Potassium	212.5 mg

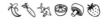

Crepes

Crepes are easy to make, and your children will have tremendous fun flipping them! This recipe uses a 50/50 mixture of whole-wheat and white flour to boost the vitamin, iron, and fiber content. The eggs and milk are good sources of protein, and the fruit fillings provide extra vitamins.

½ cup all-purpose flour

½ cup whole-wheat flour

2 large eggs

1 cup milk

Possible crepe fillings: sliced banana mixed with a little honey, sliced strawberries mixed with strawberry yogurt, apple purée and raisins, raspberries lightly mashed with a little sugar, sliced mango, fresh or canned pineapple, etc.

Process all ingredients, except crepe fillings, in a blender or food processor until smooth. Or, mix the flours in a bowl. Make a well in the center. Beat the egg and milk separately, and gradually add to the flour, beating to make a smooth batter.

Heat greased crepe pan or small skillet over medium heat. Pour enough batter into the skillet to coat the pan thinly and cook for 1–2 minutes until golden brown on the bottom. Turn the crepe and cook until browned on the bottom, 30–60 seconds. Turn out on a plate; cover and keep warm while you make the other crepes. Serve with any of the fillings.

Makes 10–12 crepes (10 servings).

PER SERVING: 70.0 calories / 3.5 g protein / 10.3 g carbohydrate / 0.9 g fiber / 1.6 g total fat / 0.6 g saturated fat / 44.3 mg cholesterol / 24.4 mg sodium

NUTRITIONAL ANALYSIS PER SERVING

Vitamin A	28.3	RE	Vitamin D	0.4 µg	Thiamin (B-1)	0.1 mg	Vitamin E	0.2 mg
Riboflavin (B-2)	0.1	mg	Calcium	36.8 mg	Niacin	0.8 mg	Iron	0.7 mg
Vitamin B-6	0.0	mg	Phosphorus	69.5 mg	Vitamin B-12	0.2 µg	Magnesium	13.5 mg
Folate (total)	20.0	µg	Zinc	0.4 mg	Vitamin C	0.0 mg	Potassium	81.0 mg

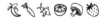

Crunchy Apple Crumble

This recipe provides a delicious way of adding extra fruit to your children's diet. The whole-wheat flour provides iron, fiber, and B vitamins, and the almonds provide protein and calcium.

1½ pounds cooking apples, peeled and sliced

2 ounces raisins

¼ cup sugar

½ teaspoon ground cinnamon

¼ cup water

½ cup all-purpose flour

½ cup whole-wheat flour

4 tablespoons butter or margarine, cold

¼ cup packed brown sugar

1 ounce toasted almonds or other nuts (walnuts, pecans, hazelnuts), chopped

Preheat the oven to 375°F.

Place the apples, raisins, sugar, and cinnamon in a deep baking dish. Toss and pour the water over the mixture.

Measure the flours into a bowl and cut in the butter with pastry blender until the mixture resembles coarse crumbs. Mix in the sugar and almonds. Sprinkle over the apples. Bake, uncovered, for 20–25 minutes, or until browned.

Makes 4 servings.

Variations

Substitute 1½ pounds peeled, sliced prepared fruit for the apples. Try the following: apples and blackberries, chopped rhubarb and sugar, fresh or canned apricots, pears and raspberries, fresh plums, blueberries, pears and bananas, etc.

PER SERVING: 473.3 calories / 6.2 g protein / 82.7 g carbohydrate / 7.5 g fiber / 15.9 g total fat / 7.7 g saturated fat / 30.5 mg cholesterol / 91.5 mg sodium

NUTRITIONAL ANALYSIS PER SERVING

Vitamin A	79.1 RE	Vitamin D	0.2 µg	Thiamin (B-1)	0.3 mg	Vitamin E	2.9 mg
Riboflavin (B-2)	0.2 mg	Calcium	60.2 mg	Niacin	2.4 mg	Iron	2.4 mg
Vitamin B-6	0.2 mg	Phosphorus	140.5 mg	Vitamin B-12	0.0 µg	Magnesium	60.4 mg
Folate (total)	43.3 µg	Zinc	0.9 mg	Vitamin C	7.6 mg	Potassium	455.3 mg

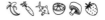

Baked Rice Pudding

This is a great-tasting, nutritious pudding, simple to make and far superior to the store-bought variety. It's rich in calcium and protein. Top with fresh fruit or fruit purée.

⅓ cup medium grain rice

2 cups milk

¼ cup sugar

Grated nutmeg

Assorted cooked or fresh
    fruit

Preheat the oven to 300°F.

Put the rice, milk, and sugar in a 1½-quart baking dish. Stir the mixture, then grate the nutmeg over the top.

Bake, uncovered for 1½ hours, or until the milk has been absorbed and there is a light-brown skin on top of the pudding. Serve with fruit.

Makes 4 servings.

PER SERVING: 165.9 calories / 5.1 g protein / 30.6 g carbohydrate / 0.2 g fiber / 2.5 g total fat / 1.6 g saturated fat / 9.8 mg cholesterol / 50.2 mg sodium

NUTRITIONAL ANALYSIS PER SERVING

Vitamin A	46.1	RE	Vitamin D	1.2 µg	Thiamin (B-1)	0.1 mg	Vitamin E	0.1	mg
Riboflavin (B-2)	0.2	mg	Calcium	144.3 mg	Niacin	4.9 mg	Iron	0.7	mg
Vitamin B-6	0.1	mg	Phosphorus	132.2 mg	Vitamin B-12	0.6 µg	Magnesium	19.1	mg
Folate (total)	43.6	µg	Zinc	0.7 mg	Vitamin C	0.2 mg	Potassium	197.2	mg

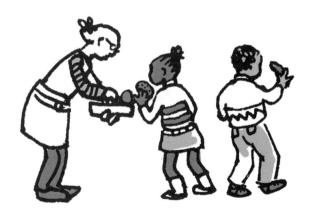

Banana Bread Pudding

This pudding is warming and comforting—great for cold days! It provides carbohydrates, fiber, protein, and calcium. You can substitute raisins or stewed plums for the bananas—delicious!

6 large slices whole-grain
    bread

3 tablespoons butter,
    softened

2 small bananas, sliced

¼ cup sugar

2 large eggs

1¾ cups milk

Ground cinnamon

Preheat the oven to 350°F.

Trim the crusts from the bread. Spread lightly with butter, and cut into quarters diagonally. Arrange one-third of the bread triangles in a lightly oiled baking dish. Arrange one of the sliced bananas on top of the bread, and repeat the layers, finishing with the bread.

Combine the sugar, eggs, and milk. Pour over the bread, then sprinkle with cinnamon. Allow to stand for 30 minutes. Bake, uncovered, for 40 minutes, or until the pudding is set and golden brown.

Makes 4 servings.

PER SERVING: 385.4 calories / 13.4 g protein / 53.2 g carbohydrate / 7.5 g fiber / 15.7 g total fat / 7.7 g saturated fat / 137.2 mg cholesterol / 275.7 mg sodium

NUTRITIONAL ANALYSIS PER SERVING

Vitamin A	146.1 RE	Vitamin D	2.7 µg	Thiamin (B-1)	0.2 mg	Vitamin E	0.7 mg
Riboflavin (B-2)	0.5 mg	Calcium	233.8 mg	Niacin	2.3 mg	Iron	1.7 mg
Vitamin B-6	0.5 mg	Phosphorus	163.6 mg	Vitamin B-12	1.0 µg	Magnesium	30.9 mg
Folate (total)	77.2 µg	Zinc	2.6 mg	Vitamin C	5.5 mg	Potassium	407.6 mg

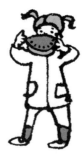

Baked Bananas

This is one of the easiest desserts. It is high in carbohydrate, low in fat, and rich in potassium and magnesium.

4 medium bananas

¼ cup water

2 tablespoons honey or
maple syrup

¼ teaspoon each ground
cinnamon and nutmeg

1½ ounces raisins

Preheat the oven to 400°F.

Cut the bananas into 1-inch chunks. Place in an oiled baking dish, and combine with the remaining ingredients. Bake, uncovered, until hot through, about 15 minutes. Serve with plain or vanilla yogurt.

Makes 4 servings.

PER SERVING: 169.8 calories / 1.7 g protein / 44.2 g carbohydrate / 3.6 g fiber / 0.5 g total fat / 0.2 g saturated fat / 0.0 mg cholesterol / 2.8 mg sodium

NUTRITIONAL ANALYSIS PER SERVING

Vitamin A	9.6 RE	Vitamin D	0.0 µg	Thiamin (B-1)	0.0 mg	Vitamin E	0.4 mg
Riboflavin (B-2)	0.1 mg	Calcium	13.9 mg	Niacin	0.9 mg	Iron	0.6 mg
Vitamin B-6	0.5 mg	Phosphorus	37.5 mg	Vitamin B-12	0.0 µg	Magnesium	35.8 mg
Folate (total)	24.5 µg	Zinc	0.2 mg	Vitamin C	10.6 mg	Potassium	508.7 mg

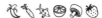

Yogurt and Fruit Pudding

A nutritious everyday pudding that counts towards the 5 servings of fruits and vegetables recommended for children.

1 carton (4 to 6 ounces) fruit
yogurt

4 ounces fresh or stewed
fruit (mango,
strawberries, blueberries,
raspberries, peaches,
bananas)

1 tablespoon toasted
slivered almonds or
hazelnuts

Spoon half of the yogurt into a sundae glass or small dish. Top with half of the fruit, followed by another layer of yogurt. Top with the remaining fruit and nuts.

Makes 1 serving.

PER SERVING: 236.3 calories / 7.2 g protein / 42.5 g carbohydrate / 3.0 g fiber / 5.6 g total fat / 1.2 g saturated fat / 4.5 mg cholesterol / 68.1 mg sodium

NUTRITIONAL ANALYSIS PER SERVING

Vitamin A	453.7 RE	Vitamin D	0.0 µg	Thiamin (B-1)	0.1 mg	Vitamin E	3.4 mg
Riboflavin (B-2)	0.3 mg	Calcium	203.9 mg	Niacin	1.1 mg	Iron	0.6 mg
Vitamin B-6	0.2 mg	Phosphorus	185.9 mg	Vitamin B-12	0.5 µg	Magnesium	49.6 mg
Folate (total)	28.4 µg	Zinc	1.2 mg	Vitamin C	32.2 mg	Potassium	457.2 mg

Cherry Clafouti

This baked French custard is low in fat and is a good source of protein, vitamins, and calcium. You can substitute other fresh or canned fruit, such as apricots, peaches, plums, or pears, for the cherries.

½ cup all-purpose flour

⅓ cup sugar

2 large eggs

1½ cups milk

1 can (14 ounces) black cherries, drained

Pinch of grated nutmeg

Preheat the oven to 400°F.

Process the flour, sugar, eggs, and milk in a blender or food processor until smooth. Arrange the cherries evenly in the bottom of an oiled baking dish. Pour the batter over and sprinkle the top with nutmeg. Bake, uncovered, for 40–45 minutes, or until the custard is set.

Makes 4 servings.

PER SERVING: 305.7 calories / 8.5 g protein / 57.7 g carbohydrate / 1.2 g fiber / 4.4 g total fat / 1.9 g saturated fat / 113.1 mg cholesterol / 80.3 mg sodium

NUTRITIONAL ANALYSIS PER SERVING

Vitamin A	82.3 RE	Vitamin D	1.2 µg	Thiamin (B-1)	0.2 mg	Vitamin E	0.3 mg
Riboflavin (B-2)	0.4 mg	Calcium	122.8 mg	Niacin	1.0 mg	Iron	1.5 mg
Vitamin B-6	0.1 mg	Phosphorus	150.6 mg	Vitamin B-12	0.7 µg	Magnesium	16.5 mg
Folate (total)	44.9 µg	Zinc	0.8 mg	Vitamin C	1.1 mg	Potassium	389.2 mg

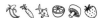

Banana and Nut Fool

This creamy pudding is a great source of protein, calcium, and potassium.

2 medium bananas

Juice of ½ lemon

1 carton (6 ounces) plain or vanilla yogurt

2 ounces chopped walnuts or pistachios

Mash the bananas with a fork and combine with the lemon juice. Stir in the yogurt and nuts, and spoon into 4 bowls.

Makes 4 servings.

PER SERVING: 175.8 calories / 5.1 g protein / 19.7 g carbohydrate / 2.5 g fiber / 10.1 g total fat / 1.4 g saturated fat / 2.6 mg cholesterol / 30.8 mg sodium

NUTRITIONAL ANALYSIS PER SERVING

Vitamin A	12.4 RE	Vitamin D	0.0 µg	Thiamin (B-1)	0.1 mg	Vitamin E	0.6 mg
Riboflavin (B-2)	0.2 mg	Calcium	95.7 mg	Niacin	0.6 mg	Iron	0.6 mg
Vitamin B-6	0.3 mg	Phosphorus	124.2 mg	Vitamin B-12	0.2 µg	Magnesium	46.5 mg
Folate (total)	32.4 µg	Zinc	0.9 mg	Vitamin C	12.7 mg	Potassium	392.1 mg

Summer Fruit Salad 1

Try to combine fruits with contrasting colors. This helps to make it more appealing to children. Remember, all types of berries (strawberries, raspberries, blackberries, blueberries) are rich in vitamin C. Orange-colored fruit, such as cantaloupe, apricots, and nectarines, are rich in beta-carotene. And the more intensely colored the fruit, the higher the antioxidant content.

4 ounces strawberries or
    other berries

4 small slices cantaloupe,
    diced

1 nectarine, chopped

¾ cup unsweetened
    pineapple, orange, or
    apple juice

1 cup vanilla yogurt

Combine the fruit and fruit juice in a bowl. Spoon into individual bowls and top with vanilla yogurt.
    Makes 4 servings.

PER SERVING: 122.4 calories / 4.2 g protein / 25.5 g carbohydrate / 1.8 g fiber / 1.1 g total fat / 0.5 g saturated fat / 3.1 mg cholesterol / 50.6 mg sodium

NUTRITIONAL ANALYSIS PER SERVING

Vitamin A	224.0 RE	Vitamin D	0.0 µg	Thiamin (B-1)	0.1 mg	Vitamin E	0.5 mg
Riboflavin (B-2)	0.2 mg	Calcium	124.6 mg	Niacin	1.1 mg	Iron	0.5 mg
Vitamin B-6	0.1 mg	Phosphorus	110.9 mg	Vitamin B-12	0.3 µg	Magnesium	29.7 mg
Folate (total)	38.4 µg	Zinc	0.8 mg	Vitamin C	45.7 mg	Potassium	466.2 mg

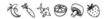

Summer Fruit Salad 2

8 ounces raspberries

8 ounces green grapes

¾ cup apple juice

1 cup vanilla yogurt

Combine the grapes and apple juice in a bowl. Spoon into individual bowls and top with vanilla yogurt.
    Makes 4 servings.

PER SERVING: 142.5 calories / 4.1 g protein / 30.9 g carbohydrate / 4.2 g fiber / 1.3 g total fat / 0.5 g saturated fat / 3.1 mg cholesterol / 43.5 mg sodium

NUTRITIONAL ANALYSIS PER SERVING

Vitamin A	19.3 RE	Vitamin D	0.0 µg	Thiamin (B-1)	0.1 mg	Vitamin E	0.7 mg
Riboflavin (B-2)	0.2 mg	Calcium	127.8 mg	Niacin	0.6 mg	Iron	0.8 mg
Vitamin B-6	0.1 mg	Phosphorus	113.7 mg	Vitamin B-12	0.3 µg	Magnesium	27.6 mg
Folate (total)	19.8 µg	Zinc	0.8 mg	Vitamin C	21.9 mg	Potassium	383.4 mg

Winter Fruit Salad

Make the most of vitamin C–rich citrus fruit by combining with other seasonal fruits such as apples and pears.

1 medium apple, thinly sliced

2 tangerines, peeled,
    sectioned

2 kiwi fruit, peeled and sliced

¾ cup orange juice

1 cup vanilla yogurt

Combine the fruit and orange juice in a bowl. Spoon into individual bowls and top with vanilla yogurt.
    Makes 4 servings.

PER SERVING: 136.4 calories / 4.2 g protein / 29.2 g carbohydrate / 2.8 g fiber / 1.2 g total fat / 0.5 g saturated fat / 3.1 mg cholesterol / 43.2 mg sodium

NUTRITIONAL ANALYSIS PER SERVING

Vitamin A	64.5 RE	Vitamin D	0.0 µg	Thiamin (B-1)	0.1 mg	Vitamin E	0.7 mg
Riboflavin (B-2)	0.2 mg	Calcium	140.4 mg	Niacin	0.6 mg	Iron	0.4 mg
Vitamin B-6	0.1 mg	Phosphorus	115.7 mg	Vitamin B-12	0.3 µg	Magnesium	28.1 mg
Folate (total)	37.9 µg	Zinc	0.6 mg	Vitamin C	71.8 mg	Potassium	452.3 mg

CHAPTER 20

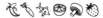

Kids' Snacks

Hummus

Hummus makes a great high-protein snack. Serve as a dip with crudités to encourage children to eat more vegetables. It also makes a satisfying sandwich filling or baked potato topping.

2 cans (15 ounces each) chickpeas, undrained

2 garlic cloves

2 tablespoons olive oil

¼ cup tahini (sesame seed paste)

Juice of 1 lemon

Pinch of paprika

⅛ teaspoon freshly ground black pepper

6–8 pitas, cut into triangles

Drain chickpeas and rinse, reserving liquid. Process chickpeas and the remaining ingredients, except pita triangles, with enough of the reserved chickpea liquid to make a creamy consistency. Chill in the fridge and serve with pita triangles.

Makes about 1 pint (4 servings).

PER SERVING: 632.9 calories / 22.3 g protein / 99.7 g carbohydrate / 11.7 g fiber / 18.6 g total fat / 2.3 g saturated fat / 0.0 mg cholesterol / 1076.6 mg sodium

NUTRITIONAL ANALYSIS PER SERVING

Vitamin A	9.6	RE	Vitamin D	0.0 µg	Thiamin (B-1)	0.8 mg	Vitamin E	1.2	mg
Riboflavin (B-2)	0.4	mg	Calcium	243.4 mg	Niacin	5.1 mg	Iron	6.3	mg
Vitamin B-6	1.1	mg	Phosphorus	396.1 mg	Vitamin B-12	0.0 µg	Magnesium	100.2	mg
Folate (total)	179.2	µg	Zinc	3.7 mg	Vitamin C	16.3 mg	Potassium	564.5	mg

Apple Muffins

These healthy muffins are excellent for lunchboxes and after-school snacks. The apples boost the fiber and vitamin content of the muffins.

¼ cup canola oil

⅔ cup packed brown sugar

2 large eggs

½ cup milk

1 teaspoon vanilla extract

2 small apples, peeled, cored, and grated

1¾ cups self-rising flour

Preheat the oven to 375°F.

Combine the oil, sugar, eggs, milk, and vanilla extract in a bowl. Stir in the grated apples and flour. Spoon the mixture into greased muffin tins. Bake for 15–20 minutes, or until golden brown.

Makes 12 muffins.

PER SERVING: 181.0 calories / 3.2 g protein / 29.2 g carbohydrate / 1.0 g fiber / 5.8 g total fat / 0.7 g saturated fat / 36.1 mg cholesterol / 252.4 mg sodium

NUTRITIONAL ANALYSIS PER SERVING

Vitamin A	20.9 RE	Vitamin D	0.2 µg	Thiamin (B-1)	0.1 mg	Vitamin E	1.1 mg
Riboflavin (B-2)	0.1 mg	Calcium	89.7 mg	Niacin	1.1 mg	Iron	1.3 mg
Vitamin B-6	0.0 mg	Phosphorus	139.2 mg	Vitamin B-12	0.2 µg	Magnesium	10.3 mg
Folate (total)	41.0 µg	Zinc	0.3 mg	Vitamin C	1.1 mg	Potassium	116.5 mg

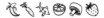

Fruit Muffins

These are perfect snacks for refueling after sports. They are made with whole-wheat flour, which is rich in fiber, iron, and B vitamins, and raisins, a great source of antioxidants. Make sure you pop one in your child's backpack.

2 cups self-rising flour (a blend of 1 cup white and 1 cup wheat)

Pinch of salt

3 tablespoons packed brown sugar

2 tablespoons canola oil

1 large egg

1¾ cups milk

3 ounces raisins

Preheat the oven to 425°F.

Mix the flour and salt in a bowl. Add the sugar, oil, egg, and milk. Mix well. Stir in the raisins. Spoon into greased muffin tins and bake for 15–20 minutes, or until golden brown.

Makes 12 muffins (12 servings).

PER SERVING: 151.9 calories / 4.0 g protein / 26.1 g carbohydrate / 0.8 g fiber / 3.6 g total fat / 0.8 g saturated fat / 20.5 mg cholesterol / 287.1 mg sodium

NUTRITIONAL ANALYSIS PER SERVING

Vitamin A	21.5 RE	Vitamin D	0.4 µg	Thiamin (B-1)	0.2 mg	Vitamin E	0.6 mg
Riboflavin (B-2)	0.2 mg	Calcium	120.7 mg	Niacin	1.3 mg	Iron	1.3 mg
Vitamin B-6	0.0 mg	Phosphorus	176.3 mg	Vitamin B-12	0.2 µg	Magnesium	11.6 mg
Folate (total)	45.0 µg	Zinc	0.4 mg	Vitamin C	0.2 mg	Potassium	149.8 mg

Banana Muffins

These banana muffins make great after-sport or after-school snacks.

2 large ripe bananas, mashed

½ cup packed brown sugar

¼ cup canola oil

1 large egg

½ cup milk

1⅔ cups self-rising flour

Pinch of salt

½ teaspoon grated nutmeg

Preheat the oven to 375°F.

Mix the bananas, sugar, and oil in large bowl. Beat in the egg and milk. Stir in the flour, salt, and nutmeg. Spoon into greased muffin tins and bake for 15–20 minutes, or until golden brown.

Makes 12 muffins (12 servings).

PER SERVING: 165.3 calories / 2.8 g protein / 26.9 g carbohydrate / 1.0 g fiber / 5.4 g total fat / 0.7 g saturated fat / 18.4 mg cholesterol / 234.3 mg sodium

NUTRITIONAL ANALYSIS PER SERVING

Vitamin A	13.4 RE	Vitamin D	0.2 µg	Thiamin (B-1)	0.1 mg	Vitamin E	1.1 mg
Riboflavin (B-2)	0.1 mg	Calcium	81.7 mg	Niacin	1.2 mg	Iron	1.1 mg
Vitamin B-6	0.1 mg	Phosphorus	127.4 mg	Vitamin B-12	0.1 µg	Magnesium	13.1 mg
Folate (total)	40.6 µg	Zinc	0.2 mg	Vitamin C	1.7 mg	Potassium	144.8 mg

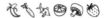

Banana Loaf

This popular cake is made with whole-wheat flour, brown sugar, and canola oil, instead of the usual white flour, white sugar, and butter.

1¾ cups self-rising whole-wheat flour

⅔ cup packed brown sugar

Pinch of salt

½ teaspoon each ground nutmeg and cinnamon

2 large ripe bananas

¾ cup orange juice

2 large eggs

¼ cup canola oil

Preheat the oven to 325°F.

Mix the flour, sugar, salt, and spices in a bowl. Mash the bananas with the orange juice. Combine the mashed banana mixture, eggs, and oil with the flour mixture.

Spoon into an oiled 9 x 5–inch loaf pan. Bake until toothpick inserted in center of bread comes out clean, about 1 hour. Cool on wire rack 10 minutes; remove bread and cool.

Makes 12 slices (12 servings).

PER SERVING: 188.2 calories / 3.2 g protein / 31.7 g carbohydrate / 1.1 g fiber / 5.7 g total fat / 0.7 g saturated fat / 32.3 mg cholesterol / 248.3 mg sodium

NUTRITIONAL ANALYSIS PER SERVING

Vitamin A	20.6 RE	Vitamin D	0.1 µg	Thiamin (B-1)	0.2 mg	Vitamin E	1.1 mg
Riboflavin (B-2)	0.1 mg	Calcium	80.5 mg	Niacin	1.3 mg	Iron	1.4 mg
Vitamin B-6	0.1 mg	Phosphorus	134.3 mg	Vitamin B-12	0.1 µg	Magnesium	15.2 mg
Folate (total)	48.5 µg	Zinc	0.3 mg	Vitamin C	9.5 mg	Potassium	178.3 mg

Apple Spice Cake

This recipe is a great way of adding extra fruit to your children's diet. The grated apple and the canola oil make this cake deliciously moist.

2½ cups self-rising flour (half white, half whole-wheat)

⅔ cup packed brown sugar

1 teaspoon ground cinnamon

2 small cooking apples, peeled and grated

¼ cup canola oil

2 large eggs

½ cup milk

Powdered sugar

Preheat the oven to 325°F.

Mix the flour, sugar, and cinnamon in a bowl. Add the grated apples, canola oil, eggs, and milk, and combine well. Spoon batter into a greased and floured 9 x 5–inch loaf pan. Bake until toothpick inserted in center comes out clean, 1–1¼ hours. Cool on wire rack 10 minutes; remove cake and cool. Sprinkle with powdered sugar.

Makes 12 slices (12 servings).

PER SERVING: 208.2 calories / 4.0 g protein / 35.1 g carbohydrate / 1.4 g fiber / 5.9 g total fat / 0.8 g saturated fat / 36.1 mg cholesterol / 351.6 mg sodium

NUTRITIONAL ANALYSIS PER SERVING

Vitamin A	21.0 RE	Vitamin D	0.2 µg	Thiamin (B-1)	0.2 mg	Vitamin E	1.1 mg
Riboflavin (B-2)	0.2 mg	Calcium	118.5 mg	Niacin	1.6 mg	Iron	1.7 mg
Vitamin B-6	0.0 mg	Phosphorus	185.8 mg	Vitamin B-12	0.2 µg	Magnesium	11.9 mg
Folate (total)	56.3 µg	Zinc	0.3 mg	Vitamin C	1.1 mg	Potassium	126.6 mg

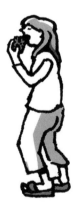

Carrot Cake

Traditional carrot cakes have a very high oil/fat and sugar content and are smothered in cream cheese. This version is lower in fat and sugar, and is made with grated apples and carrots.

1¾ cups self-rising flour (half white, half whole wheat)

Pinch of salt

1 teaspoon ground cinnamon

1 teaspoon ground nutmeg

⅔ cup packed brown sugar

2 large eggs

1 teaspoon vanilla extract

3 carrots, shredded

2 apples, shredded

¼ cup canola oil

½ cup milk

Powdered sugar

Preheat the oven to 325°F.

Mix the flour, salt, spices, and sugar in a bowl. Stir in the eggs, vanilla, carrots, apples, oil, and milk.

Line an 8-inch round cake pan with waxed paper or parchment paper. Spoon in the cake batter. Bake until toothpick inserted in center of cake comes out clean, 30 to 40 minutes. Cool cake in pan on wire rack 10 minutes; remove cake, cool, and peel off parchment. Sprinkle with powdered sugar.

Makes 16 slices (16 servings).

PER SERVING: 141.5 calories / 2.6 g protein / 23.2 g carbohydrate / 1.2 g fiber / 4.4 g total fat / 0.6 g saturated fat / 27.0 mg cholesterol / 197.2 mg sodium

NUTRITIONAL ANALYSIS PER SERVING

Vitamin A	337.5 RE	Vitamin D	0.2 µg	Thiamin (B-1)	0.1 mg	Vitamin E	0.9 mg
Riboflavin (B-2)	0.1 mg	Calcium	73.1 mg	Niacin	0.9 mg	Iron	1.0 mg
Vitamin B-6	0.0 mg	Phosphorus	108.8 mg	Vitamin B-12	0.1 µg	Magnesium	9.4 mg
Folate (total)	33.0 µg	Zinc	0.2 mg	Vitamin C	1.5 mg	Potassium	125.1 mg

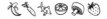

Fruit Cake

The dried fruit and grated apple add plenty of vitamins and fiber to this cake. It makes a nutritious snack anytime.

1¾ cups self rising flour

½ cup packed brown sugar

1 teaspoon ground
  cinnamon

2 large eggs

¼ cup canola oil

1 teaspoon vanilla extract

8 ounces mixed dried fruit,
  chopped (raisins, dried
  apricots, dried apples,
  dried pineapple)

1 small apple, grated

⅓ cup milk

Preheat the oven to 325°F.

Mix the flour, sugar, and cinnamon in a bowl. Make a well in the center of the dry ingredients, and add the eggs, oil, vanilla, dried fruit, apple, and milk. Mix well.

Spoon into a greased and floured 8-inch round or square baking pan and bake until skewer inserted in center of cake comes out clean, 1¼–1½ hours. Cool on wire rack 15 minutes; remove from pan and cool.

Makes 16 slices (16 servings).

PER SERVING: 160.0 calories / 2.8 g protein / 28.5 g carbohydrate / 1.4 g fiber / 4.3 g total fat / 0.5 g saturated fat / 0.0 mg cholesterol / 188.8 mg sodium

NUTRITIONAL ANALYSIS PER SERVING

Vitamin A	65.7	RE	Vitamin D	0.1	µg	Thiamin (B-1)	0.1	mg	Vitamin E	1.2	mg
Riboflavin (B-2)	0.1	mg	Calcium	71.1	mg	Niacin	1.1	mg	Iron	1.3	mg
Vitamin B-6	0.0	mg	Phosphorus	112.8	mg	Vitamin B-12	0.1	µg	Magnesium	11.0	mg
Folate (total)	31.4	µg	Zinc	0.2	mg	Vitamin C	0.7	mg	Potassium	202.5	mg

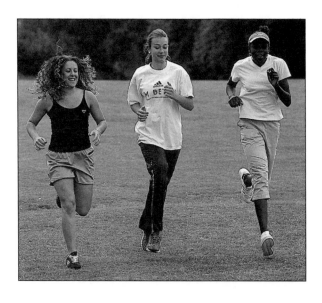

Ginger Spice Cake

This delicious cake is lower in fat and sugar than the traditional version, yet is deliciously moist as it is made with canola oil, which is rich in healthy monounsaturates.

1⅔ cups all-purpose flour

1 teaspoon baking soda

1 teaspoon ground
   cinnamon

1 teaspoon ground ginger

1 teaspoon ground cloves

1 large egg

⅔ cup packed brown sugar

¼ cup canola oil

¾ cup low-fat plain yogurt

2–3 tablespoons chopped
   pecans

Preheat the oven to 325°F.

Mix the flour, baking soda, and spices in a bowl. Whisk the egg, sugar, and oil together until light and fluffy; stir in the yogurt and mix well. Gently fold in the flour and spice mixture.

Spoon batter into greased and floured 9 x 5–inch loaf pan and sprinkle with the chopped nuts. Bake until toothpick inserted in center of cake comes out clean, about 45 minutes. Cool on wire rack 10 minutes; remove cake and cool.

Makes 10 slices (10 servings).

PER SERVING: 207.3 calories / 3.8 g protein / 31.7 g carbohydrate / 0.9 g fiber / 7.5 g total fat / 0.9 g saturated fat / 22.3 mg cholesterol / 416.7 mg sodium

NUTRITIONAL ANALYSIS PER SERVING

Vitamin A	12.8 RE	Vitamin D	0.1 µg	Thiamin (B-1)	0.2 mg	Vitamin E	1.3 mg
Riboflavin (B-2)	0.2 mg	Calcium	124.5 mg	Niacin	1.3 mg	Iron	1.5 mg
Vitamin B-6	0.0 mg	Phosphorus	167.6 mg	Vitamin B-12	0.2 µg	Magnesium	14.6 mg
Folate (total)	46.0 µg	Zinc	0.5 mg	Vitamin C	0.4 mg	Potassium	137.7 mg

Whole-Wheat Raisin Cookies

These cookies are far healthier than commercial ones. They are lower in sugar and higher in fiber.

1 ¾ cups whole-wheat flour

3 tablespoons packed brown sugar

3 ounces raisins

2 tablespoons canola oil

1 large egg

¼ cup milk

Preheat the oven to 350°F.

Combine the flour, sugar, and raisins in a bowl. Add the oil, egg, and milk, and mix to make a stiff dough. Place spoonfuls of the mixture onto a lightly oiled cookie sheet. Bake for 12–15 minutes, or until golden brown. Cool on wire racks.

Makes 20 cookies (20 servings).

PER SERVING: 73.3 calories / 2.0 g protein / 13.2 g carbohydrate / 1.4 g fiber / 1.9 g total fat / 0.2 g saturated fat / 10.8 mg cholesterol / 6.5 mg sodium

NUTRITIONAL ANALYSIS PER SERVING

Vitamin A	6.0 RE	Vitamin D	0.1 µg	Thiamin (B-1)	0.1 mg	Vitamin E	0.5 mg
Riboflavin (B-2)	0.0 mg	Calcium	12.3 mg	Niacin	0.7 mg	Iron	0.6 mg
Vitamin B-6	0.0 mg	Phosphorus	48.7 mg	Vitamin B-12	0.0 µg	Magnesium	17.1 mg
Folate (total)	6.2 µg	Zinc	0.4 mg	Vitamin C	0.1 mg	Potassium	89.4 mg

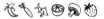

Apricot Bars

Dried apricots are packed with beta-carotene, a powerful antioxidant that's also good for the skin.

1 cup self-rising flour

⅓ cup sugar

4 ounces dried apricots

⅓ cup orange juice

2 large eggs

4 ounces raisins

Preheat the oven to 350°F.

Mix the flour and sugar in a bowl. Process the apricots and juice in a blender or food processor until smooth. Mix apricot purée into flour mixture together with the eggs and raisins. Spoon the mixture into a greased and floured 8-inch baking pan. Bake for 30–35 minutes, or until golden brown. Cool on wire rack. Cut into bars.

Makes 8 bars (8 servings).

PER SERVING: 185.8 calories / 4.1 g protein / 40.9 g carbohydrate / 2.0 g fiber / 1.6 g total fat / 0.4 g saturated fat / 52.9 mg cholesterol / 219.0 mg sodium

NUTRITIONAL ANALYSIS PER SERVING

Vitamin A	128.7 RE	Vitamin D	0.2 µg	Thiamin (B-1)	0.1 mg	Vitamin E	0.9 mg
Riboflavin (B-2)	0.2 mg	Calcium	75.5 mg	Niacin	1.4 mg	Iron	1.6 mg
Vitamin B-6	0.1 mg	Phosphorus	143.0 mg	Vitamin B-12	0.1 µg	Magnesium	14.7 mg
Folate (total)	41.7 µg	Zinc	0.3 mg	Vitamin C	5.6 mg	Potassium	327.8 mg

Cereal Bars

These highly nutritious bars are made from oats and granola, which provide slow-release sustained energy. They are lower in fat than commercial cereal bars.

6 ounces uncooked oats

3 ounces granola cereal (avoid the added sugar variety)

5 ounces mixed dried fruit

3 tablespoons honey

2 egg whites

¾ cup apple juice

Preheat the oven to 350°F.

Combine the oats, granola, and dried fruit in a bowl. Warm the honey in a small saucepan until it is thin; mix into oats mixture. Stir in egg whites and apple juice.

Press the mixture into a lightly oiled 9-inch baking pan. Bake for 20–25 minutes, until golden. Cool on wire rack; cut into bars.

Makes 12 bars (12 servings).

PER SERVING: 144.4 calories / 4.2 g protein / 27.3 g carbohydrate / 3.0 g fiber / 2.7 g total fat / 0.5 g saturated fat / 0.0 mg cholesterol / 52.8 mg sodium

NUTRITIONAL ANALYSIS PER SERVING

Vitamin A	252.7 RE	Vitamin D	0.0 μg	Thiamin (B-1)	0.2 mg	Vitamin E	1.1 mg
Riboflavin (B-2)	0.2 mg	Calcium	63.1 mg	Niacin	2.4 mg	Iron	4.8 mg
Vitamin B-6	0.3 mg	Phosphorus	94.7 mg	Vitamin B-12	0.0 μg	Magnesium	39.3 mg
Folate (total)	47.6 μg	Zinc	0.8 mg	Vitamin C	0.5 mg	Potassium	220.1 mg

CHAPTER 21

Delicious Drinks

Banana Milkshake

This simple, nutritious shake makes a great refueling drink at any time of the day.

1 cup milk

1 small ripe banana, sliced

3–4 ice cubes

Process the milk and banana in blender or food processor until smooth; add ice and process until blended. Makes 2 servings.

PER SERVING: 113.5 calories / 4.7 g protein / 19.2 g carbohydrate / 1.5 g fiber / 2.6 g total fat / 1.6 g saturated fat / 9.8 mg cholesterol / 50.6 mg sodium

NUTRITIONAL ANALYSIS PER SERVING

Vitamin A	50.8 RE	Vitamin D	1.2 µg	Thiamin (B-1)	0.1 mg	Vitamin E	0.2 mg
Riboflavin (B-2)	0.3 mg	Calcium	145.7 mg	Niacin	0.5 mg	Iron	0.2 mg
Vitamin B-6	0.3 mg	Phosphorus	127.7 mg	Vitamin B-12	0.6 µg	Magnesium	29.3 mg
Folate (total)	17.9 µg	Zinc	0.6 mg	Vitamin C	5.4 mg	Potassium	394.2 mg

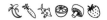

Strawberry Milkshake

Strawberries are an excellent source of vitamin C.

½ cup milk

1 carton (6 ounces) low-fat
strawberry yogurt

1 handful of strawberries

3–4 ice cubes

Process the milk, yogurt, and strawberries in a blender or food processor until smooth; add ice and process until blended.

Makes 2 servings.

PER SERVING: 122.1 calories / 5.3 g protein / 20.6 g carbohydrate / 0.7 g fiber / 2.1 g total fat / 1.3 g saturated fat / 9.9 mg cholesterol / 90.4 mg sodium

NUTRITIONAL ANALYSIS PER SERVING

Vitamin A	24.1	RE	Vitamin D	0.6	µg	Thiamin (B-1)	0.1	mg	Vitamin E	0.1	mg
Riboflavin (B-2)	0.3	mg	Calcium	177.2	mg	Niacin	0.2	mg	Iron	0.2	mg
Vitamin B-6	0.1	mg	Phosphorus	166.0	mg	Vitamin B-12	0.6	µg	Magnesium	11.4	mg
Folate (total)	11.7	µg	Zinc	0.3	mg	Vitamin C	23.7	mg	Potassium	311.7	mg

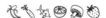

Banana Smoothie

This velvet-thick smoothie is made simply from fruit and yogurt, and doubles as a nourishing dessert.

1 large, ripe banana

1 carton (6 ounces) plain
low-fat yogurt

2 teaspoons honey

¼ cup apple juice

3–4 ice cubes

Process all the ingredients, except ice, in a blender or food processor until smooth. Add ice cubes and process until blended.

Makes 2 servings.

PER SERVING: 141.9 calories / 5.1 g protein / 28.9 g carbohydrate / 1.6 g fiber / 1.5 g total fat / 0.9 g saturated fat / 5.1 mg cholesterol / 61.3 mg sodium

NUTRITIONAL ANALYSIS PER SERVING

Vitamin A	18.3	RE	Vitamin D	0.0	µg	Thiamin (B-1)	0.1	mg	Vitamin E	2.0	mg
Riboflavin (B-2)	0.2	mg	Calcium	161.2	mg	Niacin	0.5	mg	Iron	0.4	mg
Vitamin B-6	0.3	mg	Phosphorus	137.9	mg	Vitamin B-12	0.5	µg	Magnesium	31.5	mg
Folate (total)	21.3	µg	Zinc	0.9	mg	Vitamin C	6.1	mg	Potassium	450.8	mg

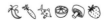

Mango and Strawberry Smoothie

Mangoes are a terrific source of beta-carotene, while strawberries provide lots of vitamin C. A super nutritious drink!

1 small mango, peeled,
    seeded

4 ounces strawberries

1 small banana

¾ cup apple juice

3–4 ice cubes

Process the fruit and apple juice in a blender or food processor until smooth. Add the ice and process until blended.

Makes 2 servings.

PER SERVING: 181.6 calories / 1.6 g protein / 42.3 g carbohydrate / 4.6 g fiber / 0.7 g total fat / 0.2 g saturated fat / 0.0 mg cholesterol / 6.0 mg sodium

NUTRITIONAL ANALYSIS PER SERVING

Vitamin A	409.0 RE	Vitamin D	0.0 µg	Thiamin (B-1) 0.1 mg	Vitamin E	1.4 mg
Riboflavin (B-2) 0.1 mg		Calcium	28.9 mg	Niacin	1.3 mg	Iron	0.9 mg
Vitamin B-6	0.4 mg	Phosphorus	44.5 mg	Vitamin B-12 0.0 µg	Magnesium	35.4 mg
Folate (total)	39.9 µg	Zinc	0.2 mg	Vitamin C	68.0 mg	Potassium	570.1 mg

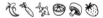

Berry Crush

This drink is bursting with vitamin C and cancer-protective phytochemicals.

8 ounces mixed fresh or
    frozen berries
    (raspberries, blueberries,
    strawberries,
    blackberries)

1 carton (6 ounces) low-fat
    raspberry yogurt

¾ cup milk

3–4 ice cubes

Process all the ingredients, except ice, in a blender or food processor until smooth. Add ice and process until blended.

Makes 2 servings.

PER SERVING: 182.6 calories / 7.1 g protein / 33.8 g carbohydrate / 5.0 g fiber / 3.1 g total fat / 1.7 g saturated fat / 12.3 mg cholesterol / 103.7 mg sodium

NUTRITIONAL ANALYSIS PER SERVING

Vitamin A	47.6 RE	Vitamin D	0.9 µg	Thiamin (B-1) 0.1 mg	Vitamin E	0.9 mg
Riboflavin (B-2) 0.4 mg		Calcium	224.7 mg	Niacin	0.7 mg	Iron	0.6 mg
Vitamin B-6	0.1 mg	Phosphorus	209.3 mg	Vitamin B-12 0.7 µg	Magnesium	25.9 mg
Folate (total)	19.9 µg	Zinc	0.7 mg	Vitamin C	21.7 mg	Potassium	426.6 mg

Tropical Delight

The mango and papaya provide lots of beta-carotene, and the lime juice is rich in vitamin C.

1 small mango, peeled and pitted

4 slices fresh or canned pineapple

1 small papaya, peeled and seeded

½ cup orange juice

Juice of 1 lime

3–4 ice cubes

Process the fruit, orange juice, and lime juice in a blender or food processor until smooth. Add ice cubes and process until blended.

Makes 2 servings.

PER SERVING: 242.8 calories / 2.9 g protein / 62.8 g carbohydrate / 7.2 g fiber / 0.8 g total fat / 0.2 g saturated fat / 0.0 mg cholesterol / 9.5 mg sodium

NUTRITIONAL ANALYSIS PER SERVING

Vitamin A	461.2 RE	Vitamin D	0.0 µg	Thiamin (B-1) 0.3 mg	Vitamin E	3.1 mg
Riboflavin (B-2) 0.2 mg	Calcium	79.8 mg	Niacin	2.2 mg	Iron	0.9 mg
Vitamin B-6	0.4 mg	Phosphorus	47.3 mg	Vitamin B-12 0.0 µg	Magnesium	54.0 mg
Folate (total) 119.1 µg	Zinc	0.4 mg	Vitamin C	223.7 mg	Potassium	905.3 mg

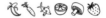

Energizer

Here's a smoothie that's full of beta-carotene, vitamin C, and potassium. It is a great energizer and immune booster.

1 small banana

1 small peach, pitted

4 ounces raspberries or strawberries

½ cup orange juice

3–4 ice cubes

Process the fruit and the orange juice in a blender or food processor until smooth. Add ice and process until blended.

Makes 2 servings.

PER SERVING: 129.0 calories / 2.2 g protein / 31.4 g carbohydrate / 6.1 g fiber / 0.8 g total fat / 0.1 g saturated fat / 0.0 mg cholesterol / 1.8 mg sodium

NUTRITIONAL ANALYSIS PER SERVING

Vitamin A	51.0 RE	Vitamin D	0.0 µg	Thiamin (B-1) 0.1 mg	Vitamin E	0.8 mg
Riboflavin (B-2) 0.1 mg	Calcium	26.9 mg	Niacin	1.4 mg	Iron	0.8 mg
Vitamin B-6	0.3 mg	Phosphorus	49.8 mg	Vitamin B-12 0.0 µg	Magnesium	39.6 mg
Folate (total) 44.3 µg	Zinc	0.4 mg	Vitamin C	54.2 mg	Potassium	513.9 mg

Strawberry and Banana Milkshake

Banana and strawberries make a delicious combination. This nutritious drink makes a great after-school or post-exercise drink.

1 small banana

4 ounces strawberries

1 carton (6 ounces) low-fat
    strawberry yogurt

½ cup milk

3–4 ice cubes

Process the fruit, yogurt, and milk in a blender or food processor until smooth. Add ice and process until blended.

Makes 2 servings.

PER SERVING: 181.2 calories / 6.0 g protein / 35.7 g carbohydrate / 2.7 g fiber / 2.3 g total fat / 1.3 g saturated fat / 9.9 mg cholesterol / 91.2 mg sodium

NUTRITIONAL ANALYSIS PER SERVING

Vitamin A	29.5 RE	Vitamin D	0.6 µg	Thiamin (B-1) 0.1 mg		Vitamin E	0.3 mg
Riboflavin (B-2)	0.3 mg	Calcium	183.4 mg	Niacin	0.7 mg	Iron	0.4 mg
Vitamin B-6	0.3 mg	Phosphorus	184.0 mg	Vitamin B-12	0.6 µg	Magnesium	30.0 mg
Folate (total)	28.5 µg	Zinc	0.4 mg	Vitamin C	41.0 mg	Potassium	554.6 mg

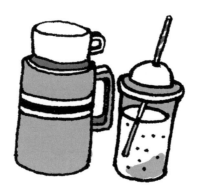

Notes

1. National Center for Health Statistics. "Prevalence of Overweight Among Children and Adolescents: United States, 1999–2002." From website of the National Center for Health Statistics, http://www.cdc.gov/nchs/products/pubs/pubd/hestats/overwght99.htm (Feb 2005).

2. Mark Lino et al., "Report Card on the Diet Quality of Children." *Family Economics and Nutrition Review* 12 (1999): 78–80. From website of the U.S. Department of Agriculture, http://www.cnpp.usda.gov/FENR/fenrv12n4/fenrv12n4p78.PDF

3. P. Tounian et al., "Presence of Increased Stiffness of the Common Carotid Artery and Endothelial Dysfunction in Severely Obese Children: A Prospective Study." *The Lancet* 358 (2001): 1400.

4. S. Dibb and L. Harris, "A Spoonful of Sugar–Television Food Advertising Aimed at Children: An International Comparative Study." *Consumers International* (1996); The Food Commission (U.K.), "Sweet Persuasion." *The Food Magazine* 9 (1990); The Food Commission (U.K.), "A Diet of Junk Food Adverts–Part Two." *The Food Magazine* 18, vol 2 (1992): 11.

5. The Food Commission *Children's Food Examined*. Food Commission (U.K.), 2000; The Food Commission, *The Food Commission Guide to Children's Food*. Food Commission (U.K.), 2000.

6. Organix, *Carrot or Chemistry?* Organix Brands (U.K.), 2002.

7. Lleana Vargas, M.D, "Type 2 Diabetes in Children and Adolescents." (Healthology, Inc., 2005). From website of *New York Daily News*, http://nydailynews.healthology.com/nydailynews/15458.htm.

8. Food and Nutrition Board, Institute of Medicine, and The National Academies. "Dietary Reference Intakes (DRIs): Recommended Intakes for Individuals, Macronutrients." *Dietary Reference Intakes Table–The Complete Set*. (National Academy of Sciences, 2002). From website of Institute of Medicine, http://www.iom.edu/Object.File/Master/21/372/0.pdf.

9. Thomas M. S. Wolever, Jennie Brand Miller, Kaye Foster-Powell, and Stephen Colagiuri, *The Glucose Revolution* (New York: Marlowe and Company, 2000); McCance and Widdowson, *The Composition of Foods*, 5th ed. (MAFF/RSC, 1991); CompEat 5 software. Nutrition Systems: Grantham.

10. R. L. Prior and G. Cao, "Analysis of Botanicals and Dietary Supplements for Antioxidant Capacity: A Review." *Journal of AOAC International* 83, vol 4 (2000): 950–6.

11.   "Prevalence of Overweight among Children and Adolescents: United States, 1999–2000." From website of the National Center for Health Statistics, http://www.cdc.gov/nchs/products/pubs/pubd/hestats/overwght99.htm.

12.   V. Burke et al., "Family Lifestyle and Parental Body Mass Index as Predictors of Body Mass Index in Australian Children: A Longitudinal Study." *International Journal of Obesity* 25 (2001): 147–57.

13.   J. K. Lake, C. Power, and T. J. Cole, "Child to Adult Body Mass Index in the 1958 British Birth Cohort: Associations with Parental Obesity." *Archive of Diseases in Childhood* 77, vol 5 (1997): 376–81.

14.   C. Bouchard, "Genetic Aspects of Human Obesity." In *Obesity*, ed. Per Bjorntorp and Bernard N. Brodoff (Philadelphia, PA: J. P. Lippincott, 1992), 343–51.

15.   Steven Dowshen, "Strength Training and Your Child." From website http://www.kidshealth.org/parent/fitness/general/strength_training.html. (2001).

16.   Gardner Merchant, *The Gardner Merchant Schools Meals Survey: What Are Our Children Eating?* (Kenley, U.K.: Gardner Merchant, 1996).

17.   "National School Lunch Program." From website of the U.S. Department of Agriculture, http://www.fns.usda.gov/cnd/Lunch/default.htm (August 2002).

18.   J. Sundgot-Borgen, "Eating Disorders in Female Athletes." *Sports Medicine* 17, vol 3 (1994): 176–88.

Resources

Online Resources

www.kidshealth.com Offers health, nutrition, and fitness advice for parents, kids, and teenagers.

www.eatright.org The website of the American Dietetic Association. Provides nutrition-related news, tips, and resources.

www.nutrition.org.uk The website of the British Nutrition Foundation. Provides information, news, and educational resources.

www.nutrio.com Includes a useful section on kids' nutrition.

www.edauk.com The website of the Eating Disorders Association (U.K.), offering information and help on all aspects of eating disorders.

www.nationaleatingdisorders.org The website of the National Eating Disorders Association, the largest nonprofit organization dedicated to eliminating eating disorders and body dissatisfaction.

www.eating-disorders.com The website of the U.S. Center for Eating Disorders. Offers information and support.

www.USDA.gov Website of the U.S. Department of Agriculture. Includes a section on children's nutrition.

Useful Addresses

National Eating Disorders Association 603 Stewart St., Suite 803
Seattle WA 98101
(206) 382-3587

American Dietetic Association 120 S. Riverside Plaza, Suite 2000
Chicago IL 60606-6995
(800) 877-1600

Recommended Reading

Joanna Blythman, *The Food Our Children Eat* (New York: HarperCollins, 1999).

Rachel Bryant-Waugh and Bryan Lask, *Eating Disorders: A Parents' Guide* (New York: Penguin, 1999).

A. H. Crisp, Neil Joughin, Christine Halek, and Carol Bowyer, *Anorexia Nervosa: The Wish to Change* (New York: Psychology Press, 1996).

Annabel Karmel, *Quick Children's Meals* (London: Ebury Press, 1997).

Janet Treasure, *Anorexia Nervosa: A Survival Guide for Families, Friends, and Sufferers* (New York: Psychology Press, 1997).

Michael Van Straten and Barbara Griggs, *Super Foods for Children* (New York: Dorling Kindersley, 2001).

Youth Sport Trust, *The Young Athlete's Handbook* (Champaign, IL: Human Kinetics, 2001).

Index

Page numbers in bold = recipe

A
acesulfame K, 12–13
additives, artificial, 12
advertising, 10–11
American Academy of Pediatrics Committee on Sports Medicine, 101
amino acids, essential (EAAs), 25, 27
androgens, 26
anemia, 52
anorexia, 113–114, 116, 118
antioxidants, 48, 58
apple: Apple Muffins, **194;** Apple Spice Cake, **196;** Crunchy Apple Crumble, **186**
Apricot Bars, **200**

B
banana: Baked Bananas, **189;** Banana and Nut Fool, **190;** Banana Bread Pudding, **188;** Banana Loaf, **195;** Banana Milkshake, **202;** Banana Muffins, **195;** Banana Smoothie, **203;** Strawberry and Banana Milkshake, **206**
beans, 19, 20, 27, 28, 32; Bean and Tuna Salad, **144;** Bean Burritos, **152;** Butter Bean and Leek Supper, **154;** Red Kidney Bean Lasagne, **150;** Spicy Bean Burgers, **172**
beta-carotenes, 48, 56
biotin, 56
blood glucose, 32–33, 62
body mass index (BMI), 81
body types, 82
boys, 31. *See also* children
breads, 27, 31–32, 106
British Health Department Agency's National Food Guide, 14
bulimia, 113–114, 116, 118
burgers, 19; Chicken Burgers, **171;** Lean Meat Burgers, **173;** Nut Burgers, **175;** Spicy Lentil Burgers, **174**

C
caffeine, 76
cakes, 22, 38; Apple Spice Cake, **196;** Carrot Cake, **197;** Fruit Cake, **198;** Ginger Spice Cake, **199**
calcium, 50–52, 56
calories, 15, 16, 37–38, 41–42, 61
candies, 22, 32, 111
carbohydrate(s), 17, 30–31, 34–36; children and, 31, 66–67; GI (glycemic index) and, 33–36; types of, 17, 32–33, 106

Carrot Cake, **197**
Cereal Bars, **201**
cereals, 27, 31–32
cheese, 18–19, 24, 27; Broccoli and Cheese Soup, **166;** Cheese and Tomato Pizza, **179;** Marvelous Macaroni and Cheese, **147;** Potato and Cheese Pie, **158**
Cherry Clafouti, **190**
chicken, 19, 27; Chicken and Mixed Pepper Risotto, **142;** Chicken and Vegetable Packets, **135;** Chicken Baked in Tomato Sauce, **131;** Chicken Burgers, **171;** Chicken Curry, **132;** Golden Baked Chicken, **134;** Homemade Chicken Nuggets, **170**
chickpeas: Chickpea and Spinach Pasta, **149;** Chickpea Hotpot, **153;** Hummus, **193**
children, 5–13, 7–9, 51; active, 59–69, 98–99; in competition/training, 61–69, 115–116; exercise and, 87–88; menu plans for, 120–130
children, overweight, 78–79, 80–84, 90; encouragement/help for, 85–87; healthier eating habits for, 88–90; lack

of physical activities and, 82, 83–84; overeating and, 82, 83; sports/weight loss and, 90–91; television and, 84, 91–92

children, underweight, 93–95; feeding, 95–98; strength training for, 100–101

Chili con Carne, **141**

cholesterol, 40, 79

competition, 61–69, 115–116

cookies, 22, 32, 38, 111; Whole-Wheat Raisin Cookies, **200**

corn, 39; Pasta with Corn and Tuna, **137**; Rice and Corn Salad, **161**

Couscous with Nuts and Vegetables, **156**

Crepes, **185**

D

Daily Values, 44

dairy, 14–16, 18–19, 23, 27–28, 38

dehydration, 70–73, 116

desserts, 12, 38; Baked Bananas as, **189**; Baked Rice Pudding as, **187**; Banana and Nut Fool as, **190**; Banana Bread Pudding as, **188**; Cherry Clafouti as, **190**; Crepes as, **185**; Crunchy Apple Crumble as, **186**; Raspberry Fool as, **184**; Summer Fruit Salads 1 and 2 as, **191**; Winter Fruit Salad as, **192**; Yogurt and Fruit Pudding as, **189**. See also snacks

diabetes, 9, 12, 32

Dietary Guidelines for Americans, 108–109

Dietary Reference Intakes (DRIs), 44

diets, 5, 7–9, 14, 78, 115

diuretics, 116

dressings, for salads; Easy Vinaigrette Dressing, **163**; general suggestions, 162; Herb Dressing, **163**

drinking, 70–72, 72–77

drinks, 76, 104; acidic, 23–24; Banana Milkshake, **202**; Banana Smoothie, **203**; Berry Crush, **204**; Energizer, **205**; Mango and Strawberry Smoothie, **204**; soft, 22, 23, 32, 76; sports, 75–77; Strawberry and Banana Milkshake, **206**; Strawberry Milkshake, **203**; Tropical Delight, **205**

DRIs. See Dietary Reference Intakes

E

EAAs. See amino acids, essential

eating, 7, 13, 102–112

eating disorders, 113–115; effects of, 116–117; prevention of, 117–119

ectomorphs, 82

EFAs. See essential fatty acids

eggs, 19, 27, 39

endomorphs, 82

energizing drink: Energizer, **205**

energy, 52, 59–69, 99, 111–112

essential fats/oils, 14–16, 20–21, 23, 39, 44

essential fatty acids (EFAs), 20–21, 39, 40

exercise, 63–65, 75–77, 87–88. See also physical activities

F

fat(s), 8, 18–19, 37–38; calories from, 15, 41–42; high, 9, 33, 62; hydrogenated, 13, 39–41; monounsaturated, 39, 40; polyunsaturated, 39, 40; saturated, 38–39, 40; trans, 40–41; unsaturated, 38–39, 40; vegetable, 38–39; vitamins and, 38. See also essential fats/oils; essential fatty acids

fatty foods, 14, 16, 38

fiber, 17, 18, 32, 33

fish, 19, 21, 27, 39; Fish Cakes, **143**

folic acids, 49, 56

food(s), 6, 8, 10, 12–13, 24, 38, 115; calcium in, 52; carbohydrate content of, 33–36; high-glycemic (fast-releasing energy), 32–33; highly refined, 32–33; organic, 46; recommended portions/servings for, 15–23; sugary, 15–16, 22–23, 62. See also Nutrition Facts; *specific types of food*

Food Guide Pyramid, 14–15, 42, 59, 103

foods, fast, 8, 19, 69; Baked Potatoes as, **180**; Cheese and Tomato Pizza as, **179**; Chicken Burgers as, **171**; Homemade Chicken Nuggets as, **170**; Lean Meat Burgers as, **173**; Mighty Root Mash as, **181**; Nut Burgers as, **175**; Oven Potato Wedges as, **182**; Pizza as, **177**; Potato Tacos as, **183**; Quick Pizza as, **178**; Spicy Bean Burgers as, **172**; Spicy Lentil Burgers as, **174**; Tomato Salsa as, **176**

fruit(s), 7, 12, 23, 32, 104–105; cakes, **196–198**; children and, 44–47; food groups, 14, 16, 44; juices, 23, 66, 75, 104; muffins, **194–195**; recommended servings/portions for, 15–16, 18, 23; salads, **191–192**; Yogurt and Fruit Pudding, **189**

G

garlic, 58

GI. See glycemic index

ginger: Ginger Spice Cake, **199**

girls, 26–27, 52, 116. See also children

glucose, 12, 30, 32–33, 62

glycemic index (GI), 33–36, 61–62
glycogen, 30
grains, 14–17, 27, 31, 39, 44

H

Harvard School of Public Health, 84
Healthy Eating Index, 7–8
hemoglobins, 43, 49, 52
heredity, 82, 94
high blood pressure, 9, 79
Hummus, **193**

I

illnesses, 8–9
iron, 17, 29, 32, 43, 52–53, 56

K

kale, curly, 58

L

lasagne: Lasagne, **140;** Red Kidney Bean Lasagne, **150**
lentils, 19, 20, 27, 32; Red Lentil Dahl, **154;** Spicy Lentil Burgers, **174**
lunches, healthy, 103, 106, 109; dairy products for, 107; fruits/vegetables for, 104–105; guidelines for, 110; treats for, 107–108, 129

M

magnesium, 32, 54, 56
Mango and Strawberry Smoothie, **204**
meals, 67–69, 108–109; main, **131–144;** meatless, **145–158;** pre-exercise, 63–64
meat(s), 19, 27–28, 38; lean, 19, 27, **173;** meatless main meals, **145–158**
menstruation, 52, 116
menu(s): for five- to ten-year-olds, 121–122, 125–126; plans for children, 120–130; for ten- to

fifteen-year-olds, 123–124, 127–128; vegetarian, 127–128. *See also specific menus*
mesomorphs, 82
Mighty Root Mash, **181**
milk, 18–19, 24, 27, 104
milkshakes: Banana Milkshake, **202;** Strawberry and Banana Milkshake, **206;** Strawberry Milkshake, **203**
minerals, 6, 17, 44–58
muffins: Apple Muffins, **194;** Banana Muffins, **195;** Fruit Muffins, **194**
muscles, 25–26, 30
mycoproteins, 19

N

National School Lunch Program, 108
niacin (vitamin B-3), 49, 56
nut(s), 19–22, 24, 27–28; allergies, 22; Nut Burgers, **175;** oil, 21, 39
Nutrition Facts, 11

O

obesity, 12, 79, 81. *See also* children, overweight
oils: coconut, 38; nut, 21, 39; palm kernel, 38; types of, 21, 39; vegetable, 38–39
omega-6, 20–21, 39, 40
omega-3, 20–21, 39, 40
Organix, 12

P

parents, 9, 79, 115
pasta, 27, 31, 32; Chickpea and Spinach Pasta, **149;** Pasta and Tuna Bake, **139;** Pasta Shells with Tomato and Peppers, **146;** Pasta Turkey Bolognese, **133;** Pasta with Corn and Tuna, **137;** Pasta with Ham and Mushroom Sauce, **138;** Vegetable and Pasta Soup, **169**

phosphorus, 56
physical activities, 8, 82, 83–84
phytochemicals, 18, 55
pizzas, **177–179**
plums, 58
potato(es), 17, 31–32, 39; Baked Potatoes, **180;** Oven Potato Wedges, **182;** Potato and Cheese Pie, **158;** Potato Salad, **160;** Potato Soup, **164;** Potato Tacos, **183**
protein, 18, 19, 25–27, 38; animal, 27; plant, 27–29; -rich foods, 14, 15–16, 19, 23, 27, 33, 44, 106; supplements, 29
prunes, 58
pyridoxine (vitamin B-6), 49, 56

Q

Quorn, 19

R

raspberries, 58; Raspberry Fool, **184**
Recommended Daily Amounts (RDAs), 44, 56
red peppers, 58
riboflavin (vitamin B-2), 48–49, 56
rice, 27, 31, 32; Baked Rice Pudding, **187**

S

salads: Bean and Tuna Salad, **144;** Coleslaw, **162;** dressings for, **162–163;** Perfect Salad, **159;** Potato Salad, **160;** Rice and Corn Salad, **161;** Summer Fruit Salads 1 and 2, **191;** Winter Fruit Salad, **192**
school, 102–112
seeds, 21, 28, 39
smoothies: Banana Smoothie, **203;** Mango and Strawberry Smoothie, **204**

snacks, 7, 12, 24, 89; after-school, 112, 129; after-sports, 130; Apple Muffins as, **194**; Apple Spice Cake as, **196**; Apricot Bars as, **200**; Banana Loaf as, **195**; Banana Muffins as, **195**; bars, 12, 38; Carrot Cake as, **197**; Cereal Bars as, **201**; during competition/training, 65–66; Fruit Cake as, **198**; Fruit Muffins as, **194**; Ginger Spice Cake as, **199**; Hummus as, **193**; for weight gain, 100; while traveling, 67–69; Whole-Wheat Raisin Cookies as, **200**. *See also* desserts
sodium, 8–9
soft drinks. *See* drinks
soups: Broccoli and Cheese Soup, **166**; Butternut Squash Soup, **167**; Carrot Soup, **168**; Potato Soup, **164**; Real Tomato Soup, **165**; Vegetable and Pasta Soup, **169**
soy, 19, 20, 27, 28, 39
spinach, 58
sports, 69, 75–77, 90–91, 130
strawberry, 58; Mango and Strawberry Smoothie, **204**; Strawberry and Banana Milkshake, **206**; Strawberry Milkshake, **203**
sucrose, 12
sugars, 9–8, 12, 15–16, 22–23, 32, 62
sunflowers, 21, 39
sweeteners, artificial, 12–13
sweets, 12, 22, 32, 111

T
teeth, 12, 23–24, 116
television, 84, 91–92
thiamin (vitamin B-1), 48, 56
Tomato Salsa, **176**
training, 61–69, 100–101
Tropical Delight, **205**
tuna: Bean and Tuna Salad, **144**; Pasta and Tuna Bake, **139**; Pasta with Corn and Tuna, **137**
turkey, 19; Pasta Turkey Bolognese, **133**

U
United States (U.S.), 7, 12, 108
U.S. Department of Agriculture, 4
U.S. Food and Nutrition Board, 26, 44

V
vegetable(s), 7–8, 31, 39, 44–47; Crispy Vegetable Gratin, **151**; food groups, 14, 16, 44; for lunches, 104–105; oils, 38–39; recommended servings/portions for, 15–16, 18; Toad-and-Vegetables-in-the-hole, **136**; Vegetable and Pasta Soup, **169**; Vegetable Korma, **155**; Vegetable Rice Feast, **156**. *See also specific vegetables*
vegetarians, 20, 27–29, 127–128, **145–158**; Bean Burritos, **152**; Butter Bean and Leak Supper, **154**; Chickpea and Spinach Pasta, **149**; Chickpea Hotpot, **153**; Couscous with Nuts and Vegetables, **157**; Crispy Vegetable Gratin, **151**; Marvelous Macaroni and Cheese, **147**; Pasta Shells with Tomato and Peppers, **146**; Penne with Cheese and Broccoli, **148**; Potato and Cheese Pie, **158**; Red Kidney Bean Lasagne, **150**; Red Lentil Dahl, **154**; Vegetable Korma, **155**; Vegetable Rice Feast, **156**; Vegetarian Spaghetti Bolognese, **145**
vitamin(s), 6, 11, 38, 43–46; A, 19, 48, 56; B, 17, 18, 32, 54; B-1 (thiamin), 48, 56; B-6 (pyridoxine), 49, 56; B-3 (niacin), 49, 56; B-12, 29, 49–50, 56; B-2 (riboflavin), 48–49, 56; C, 50, 54, 56; D, 19, 50, 56; E, 54, 56; guide to, 47–54; supplements, 54–57
vomiting, 113–114, 116

W
walking, 8, 33
water, 24, 66, 74, 104
weight loss, 90–91. *See also* children, overweight; children, underweight
Whole-Wheat Raisin Cookies, **200**

Y
yogurt, 18–19, 24, 27, 107; Yogurt and Fruit Pudding, **189**

Z
zinc, 32, 53–54, 56